Welcome to Nursing, My Name's Covid

DAVID DELANEY

authorHOUSE®

AuthorHouse™
1663 Liberty Drive
Bloomington, IN 47403
www.authorhouse.com
Phone: 833-262-8899

Published by AuthorHouse 03/02/2023

ISBN: 979-8-8230-0134-2 (sc)
ISBN: 979-8-8230-0132-8 (hc)
ISBN: 979-8-8230-0133-5 (e)

Thank you.

A warm and special thanks to my family and friends who have supported me since Day 1 on this earth and continue to do so.

An incredible thanks to Peter and Katherine who supported me on this literary endeavor since the very beginning. Without their support and enthusiasm I'm not sure I could have finished it. Their encouragement meant the world to me. Team work works.

Dedication

This Novel is dedicated to Luna Wolf who made sure everyone else was served before serving herself.

This novel is in memory of all those we lost to the pandemic too soon. May they never be forgotten.

Contents

Foreword xi

Chapter 1   February 17th, 2020 1
Chapter 2   February 18th, 2020 9
Chapter 3   February 19th 34
Chapter 4   February/March 44
Chapter 5   March 26th 56
Chapter 6   March 27th 65
Chapter 7   March 28th 71
Chapter 8   March 29th 78
Chapter 9   April 3rd 86
Chapter 10   April 4th 98
Chapter 11   April 5th-April 15th 114
Chapter 12   April 16th 122
Chapter 13   April 17th 128
Chapter 14   April 18th 141
Chapter 15   April 19th-May 25th 151
Chapter 16   May 26-July 1st 162
Chapter 17   July 2nd -August 30th 173
Chapter 18   September 192
Chapter 19   October 200
Chapter 20   November 207
Chapter 21   December 222

Chapter 22   January 239
Chapter 23   February 2021 248

March 2021 257
Gratuity List 263
Conclusion 265

Foreword

David Delaney is a brave and resilient young man. He is a skilled and compassionate nurse who fiercely advocates for his patients and profession. He is loyal and devoted to his friends and family and his commitment to sobriety. Douglas embodies a life transformed and is living proof that if you put in the work, true recovery is possible.

In his first book, *Welcome to Nursing, My Name is COVID,* David tells his story of being a newly-sober rookie nurse who is just beginning to define himself as a professional when COVID-19 Pandemic strikes. David can translate his insight from sober living into coping strategies for managing a worldwide crisis personally and professionally. David is able to analyze and change his thinking using the techniques he has picked up in the Alcohol Support Groups that he faithfully attends, choosing to find hope and positivity under dire and challenging situations. During the year of the pandemic, David comes into his own as a nurse and finds hope for the hopeless nursing home residents. He can help them overcome their personal struggles by relating them to his journey from addiction to recovery. David finds a way to inspire and motivate his elderly companions in their arduous cycle of lock downs and quarantines.

Enjoy this captivating read whether you or someone you know is in recovery; whether you or someone you know work in health care; or whether you enjoy humor or drama. There is something for everyone! *Welcome to Nursing, My Name's COVID* is a refreshing and honest read with a positive and hopeful message that the world needs right now.

I sincerely welcome you to the "frontlines".
Sophia Koury, RN, BSN

Chapter 1

February 17th, 2020

"Starting as a new nurse is just like swimming up river, with no arms, or legs... blind folded" - David Delaney

My name is David Delaney and I'm an alcoholic. It was my first day off of orientation as a new nurse—an LPN to be specific. Licensed Practical Nurse. I graduated nursing school in 2013 but was an alcoholic and the Board of Nursing knew it, and decided not to grant me my license. My license was flagged because of two DWIs. With the option to enter a program of sobriety and drug testing, I chose to continue drinking and racked up a third DWI. Six years later, after the third DWI and facing a ten year suspended driver's license, along with a six month jail sentence, I decided I should stop drinking. I called the BON and asked to enroll in their sobriety program. They accepted my enrollment and I signed a contract stating I would not use alcohol or drugs, and that I would pay the $5,000 in yearly fees and costs.

After nearly two years sober and a year and a half of compliance with the Board of Nursing's sobriety program, I began my career as a nurse. I would be in this sobriety program for a total of five years.

I got my nursing license in November of 2019 and then got hired a few months later. This would be my first job as a nurse. I was a sober alcoholic and a nurse. A good nurse at that. In addition to being a nurse, I would find that my new title would also encompass the following roles and jobs: friend, social worker, waiter, bus boy, maid, detective, actor, entertainer, life coach, secretary, body guard, security guard, peace maker advocate, translator, massage therapist, foot rubber, water boy, chef, handy man, electronic technician, and much more.

The facility that hired me was hiring anyone with a nursing license and a heartbeat. No experience, no connections, no problem. My *interview* was more of a recruitment and the *orientation* I received was nothing of the sort and prepared me in no way whatsoever for the daily grind I would endure. On top of the immense workload each nurse had each day, the pay wasn't that great. It was twenty-two dollars and change per hour... this was three dollars less than the state average for LPN's in New Jersey... two years before! No wonder no one wanted to work here.

Each nurse had anywhere from twenty to thirty residents on their unit on any given day, and their primary purpose was to give medication to them all and keep them safe. All of these resident's medications would be found on a four-and-a-half foot tall by two-and-a-half wide medication cart on wheels. The surface on the top of the cart was about two feet by sixteen inches. It was a flat but rough surface that held a fat burgundy-colored binder called the MAR (Medication Administration Record). We would prepare the medications on the flat surface and then sign each resident's flow sheets with a pen, legally documenting that the medications had been administered. Yes, it was 2020, and we were still operating on paper, seven years after a federal law was passed that required facilities, hospitals and doctor's offices to transition to electronic charting or be heftily fined. The only computer found in this facility was in the nursing station on the second floor. Anything that had to be printed or entered in the computer was relayed to someone—usually a supervisor who could access the computer and take care of it.

To the right of the cart there was a sliding tray that would come out from under the top surface and hold the bright red narcotic binder. Directly below that was the sharps container mounted to the side of the cart. Directly below that was a small trash bin, also mounted to the side of the cart. The very top drawer was only an inch and a half deep and held the stock medications, eye drops, nasal sprays, insulins—all the unimportant stuff. Well, except for the insulin. Okay, it was all important. Below the top drawer were three equal sized twelve inch deep drawers that held the resident's specific medications in "bingo cards." The nurse would pull out each card, check the medication and the dose, and pop the pill through the foil in the back of the card into a medicine cup, never touching the medication. Some residents had thirty to forty cards. It could be very time-consuming, depending on how many diagnoses a resident had. It could also be a real mess if the floor didn't have a 'regular' nurse looking after and keeping up the cart. The cart was your best friend or your worst enemy.

I worked the second shift—the 3PM-11PM shift. It was, in my opinion, easier because there were less people in the building, less distractions, less bullshit. The day shift had to put up with social workers, physical therapists, recreation therapists, family visits, nurse practitioners and doctors. I'm sure I missed a few. Second shift was a little smoother and a little calmer, although the dementia residents would begin sundowning right around dinner and that presented its own challenges. Sundowning refers to the time of day when a resident with dementia starts to *lose it.* When the sun begins to go down and evening comes, it's like Jekyll and Hide, and its actually quite fascinating unless you're the one legally responsible for said subjects. They could be pleasant and somewhat coherent during the day, but once the evening came, their wits went out the window. They became increasingly confused, agitated, and cranky. For some dementia residents their potential for violence might increase during the evenings. Luckily I was only twenty-nine. And in shape. And sober. I found out that the only way to truly prevent our residents from falling or eloping was to have eyes on them every five to fifteen minutes. That required me to sprint up and down a forty-yard hallway checking on everyone several times every hour. Did I mention I was physically fit?

My shift started at 3:00 p.m.—or 1500, as is written in the MAR. Military time is found in a lot of health care settings—one reason relevant to my practice being that there were no repeating of numbers on the clock. 4 p.m. sloppily written could be mistaken for 4 a.m. and people could be getting double-dosed. With military time, 4 p.m. was 16:00 and wasn't mistaken for the 4 o'clock in the morning time. By the time I got done receiving report from Tanya, the previous nurse, and counting the narcotics being transferred under my license, it would be around 15:30. A little too early to start my 'med-pass,' I would sit down and rest, knowing that once I started my med-pass I would not sit until I was at home, showered, and ready to go to bed.

...

At 1600 I started my med-pass at one end of the forty-yard hallway, giving out the 1600 and 1630 medications as well as the 1700 to1800 medications. I knew it was early but this was common practice and if I didn't start now, some people wouldn't get their 1700 medications until 2100 and that would certainly be unacceptable. Some residents would begin to resent me if I came too late, and they would let me have it. Other residents were more easygoing and understanding and didn't care when I came, as long as I did. Then there was the population of residents who had no concept of time and didn't even know what medication was due or when it was due.

Regardless of their cognitive status, nurses had an ethical and legal obligation to give the correct medication at the right time. Each resident had anywhere from two to ten capsules or tablets as well as eye drops and/ or nasal sprays. On top of the pills, most residents needed a 30 mL cup of a protein supplement to go along with a 30 mL cup of laxative. On top of the medicine cup shots they took, they needed a chaser—an eight-ounce dietary supplement in the form of an Ensure. On top of the chaser we had to confirm the resident could have thin liquids or if we needed to thicken everything we were about to administer. Some residents needed thickened liquid so it wouldn't go down the 'wrong pipe' and cause them to aspirate. On top of all this, we had to check blood pressure before administering anti-hypertensives. We checked blood pressures for twelve residents at 1700 and another nine BPs at 2100. The nursing tasks alone were overwhelming for anyone—even for the brightest, most hardworking and most athletic nurses. They would come to rue these medication passes and it would take everything within them to get through just one eight-hour shift!

Although some residents were easier and quicker than others, it seemed like almost every resident also needed something else done or fixed, or someone from their family had to be phoned. Picking up their TV remotes, picking up their bed remotes, finding their phone in their bed sheets, finding their eye glasses under the bed, refilling water, raising the head of the bed, but not too high. Turning the heat up, but not too hot. Pulling up the blanket but not too far up. Turning off the lights, but not all the lights. All these mundane tasks and errands had to be completed before I could move on. I didn't get into nursing to ignore and neglect the elderly and simply just pass their medications.

I suppose I should mention my nursing professor, Lily Ruffini. She said, "If you ever come across a urinal full of urine-empty it. Take the twenty-five seconds to empty it. Don't be a piece of shit." Well, I added the piece of shit part for dramatic purposes. To this day I have not ignored or walked by a single full urinal. The point I'm trying to illustrate here is that, in addition to counting, confirming, and administering approximately 200 medications and supplements to twenty-seven different humans in an eight-hour shift, anything can happen, and these residents have tons of other needs that need to be met, and these medication passes take forever and mistakes can and will always be made and things will be missed. This isn't even to mention if one of these elderly residents has difficulty breathing which needs intervention and attention, or the aforementioned fall that is inevitable, and the stack of paper work that will follow.

By 1800—two hours in, I had almost half the residents' 1700 medications completed and roughly another fourteen to go. I would finish the remaining residents in the next hour and a half. Around 2000 I could do treatments—yes, more work—which required a separate binder called a TAR. If you've been paying attention you could infer that TAR is an abbreviation for Treatment Administration Record. Or, I would start on the 2100 medication pass. I would elect for the latter and start my 2100s an hour early. The second medication pass was always a little shorter. Some residents didn't get any medications at all on the 2100 round. I could do this one in less than two hours if I focused and hurried. Not to say the 1700 medication pass didn't require complete focus and speed—without sacrificing accuracy. There were residents' lives at stake and an additional blood pressure pill could bottom out a resident and send them to heaven.

After finishing the second med-pass, I took time to eat quickly, and relieve myself in the only staff bathroom on the second floor, on the opposite side of the building. I had a quick chat with one of my orienting nurses, Florence, and gave her a quick summary of my first shift on my own. I tried to exude any confidence I had, but my feet were screaming, my soul was crying, and my brain was on fire. Still, it could be worse! We could be doing vital signs twice a shift on every resident and wearing full PPE whilst doing it!

I did the treatments that were absolutely necessary and trusted that my CNAs (Certified Nurse Assistant) were applying all the creams the residents needed after their briefs were changed. The other 'treatments' I would sign for, were things like checking that an air mattress was inflated, or that the bedside floor mattress was in place for fall risk residents, or that the bed alarm was functioning. The wounds were the most important in the TAR, and I always made sure to do every one. If you didn't do wound treatments you would quickly be found out and in trouble with the wound nurse and/or director of nursing. The bandages you placed would be signed and dated once you were done so you could keep track of how often the wound was being changed. If you signed a bandage one day, gave a report and keys to the cart to the next nurse relieving you and then returned to work the next day and see your initials and date, you knew exactly who wasn't doing their job. Meanwhile, the resident's wound could be worsening and they could be *rotting away* in bed.

Finally the day was done and I handed the keys to Rita, a nurse of seventeen years, from Jamaica.

"Me don't wanna take no keys on a dirty cart, best clean that quick before we count," she said firmly with a surprise smile at the end. She knew I was new and that I just happened to forget to clean the cart.

"Uhhh," I was processing what she had said—up to this point I hadn't used so much of my brain in the span of eight hours. "Oh right. Yeah, hold on. I'll clean that up."

She nodded and waited while I furiously cleaned. I was embarrassed but I was still relieved that I got to go home in a few minutes. We counted our narcotics and, as if she knew I'd try to leave before telling her all the happenings, she asked about report.

Embarrassment ran through all of me all over again. I fumbled with my notes and tried to remember any important or relevant information I'd come across over the past eight hours. My mind came up blank. I was so focused on getting all the meds to all the right residents, I didn't really have time for anything else. Was I a terrible nurse?

Rita sensed the panic in my body language and face and asked me to sit. We went through each resident one by one and she asked me questions. *Why didn't I do this with the nurse I relieved!?* I screamed silently to myself.

"Mr. Johnsen—did he have a bowel movement today?" she asked, looking down at the paper, waiting for an answer.

"Uh, yes he did." I wasn't entirely sure he did, but a CNA did tell me about a bowel movement from a resident in the same 260 room. There was only one other resident in that room so I had a 50% chance of being right.

"Okay, what was it like? Consistency? Color? Odor?" she asked, still looking at the paper.

"I'm actually not sure, I just know he went." *What the hell is she thinking? We're gonna go through the bowel movements of 26 residents!? You gotta be kidding me!*

"Okay, that would be good info next time so just make sure to ask the CNA. On to Mrs. Von Colson. They said last night her diaper was wet so her foley catheter might not be working. Did she have any wet diapers today?" She seemed to know I was barely staying afloat with this barrage of questions, but put me through her gauntlet anyway.

"Actually, the CNA reported no wet diapers, and the output was 450 cc, so I'm pretty sure its functioning appropriately." *Aha! I knew the answer to that one!* So that's why the CNA told me the diaper was dry and what the output was! At the time the information seemed irrelevant and just flustered me further while I was preparing tons of medications. Now, I was grateful the CNA had told me, and especially that I retained and was able to recall the information four hours later. I didn't look like a rock star with that answer but I sure felt like one for a brief moment, and thought that maybe I *do* know what the fuck is happening on my unit after all! I thought how Tanya, the nurse I'd relieved, had chosen to leave this tidbit out. As a matter of fact, she'd left every damned tidbit out! In her meek defense I didn't really ask about the happenings on the floor, but in *my* defense I didn't know what to ask about!

We went through another handful of residents. I had answers for some and I was completely lost on others. Luckily, Rita dealt with a lot of the new nurses and knew how hard it was getting started. After my half-assed report, she did say that I did a lot better than most new nurses, with the information I actually knew about my residents. That was all I needed to hear, to walk out of there with a smile on my face.

I got through the day, and although it was only one eight-hour stint, it was my first shift ever as a nurse. This was a major milestone and achievement for a degenerate and hopeless drunk.

I let Rita leave me at the desk and I sat, reflecting. I closed my eyes and meditated. I tried to think about things I'd done well, and what needed improving. As I was deep in thought I heard a loud and heavy scurrying right above my head. I looked at the dropped ceiling tile and could tell there was weight on each one—and they were sagging down. I listened as best I could and wondered what was making the noise. It wasn't coming from the third floor but rather in-between the third floor and the ceiling tiles of the second. It had to be rodents. I quickly got up from the chair and out from behind the desk—I didn't want any oversized mice falling on my head. After the disgust I felt, I decided to think back on the complement Rita had just paid me, and was left with a hopeful and optimistic feeling. I thought, it could only get better from this point on. I decided I would tell all the folks at all my different Alcohol Support Groups about my trying, exhausting, but rewarding experience as a new nurse and how none of it would have been possible without their help, and the help of Alcohol Support Groups. I decided that it would be a happy day when I shared my good news and that everyone would clap for me and congratulate me and pat me on the back. I also decided that there would be confetti and cake and maybe a ticker tape parade—okay, maybe that was going too far. I'd settle for a round of applause if it happened. They all knew my story and how I was rebuilding my life, so they'd definitely be waiting on an update.

Chapter 2

February 18th, 2020

"The expert in anything was once a beginner" - Helen Hayes

Entering my unit I was greeted by a handful of residents sitting at the corner of the hallway and the nurses station. They completely distracted my thoughts and I forgot to question the outgoing nurse, Tanya. I would soon find out the residents congregated there every day in between lunch and dinner, killing time and socializing. Meals were pretty much all they looked forward to—that, and a couple recreation activities. Every housekeeper, CNA, nurse and anyone else would have to roll their carts through the crowd—it was always a big to-do, shifting three wheelchairs, then placing them back in position. Perfectly inconvenient.

On this day, the outgoing nurse and a recreation therapist were standing there, talking to all the residents. As I got closer to the corner, Lucie Greer pointed at me and said quite animatedly, "That's him, that's the nurse!"

Oh shit, what did I do now? I really need this job, "Whats that, Lucie? What did I do?" I was used to being in trouble, so naturally I expected Lucie to accuse me of some unforgivable and heinous crime. I was ready to defend myself and scream that whatever it was, wasn't true! I braced for impact and stared Lucie down in a childish and obnoxious way.

"Oh I was just telling Marlena how *wonderful* you are and how you helped me to bed and how you rubbed my feet for so long yesterday," she said, smiling ear to ear. My first thought was: Holy shit Lucie, you almost gave me a heart attack! Followed by: *Oh, Lucie, if you only knew the 'wonderful' things I've done in my life- and I didn't rub your feet for that long.*

For some reason Marlena, the recreation therapist, had a look of skepticism that I decided to ignore. Normally my ego and I would be insulted by her reaction and harbor a resentment for her, but my Alcohol Support Group had taught me better. I was flattered and gratefully accepted the compliment and ignored Marlena's shallow skepticism.

"Aw, thank you Lucie, I appreciate that!" I said quietly, lowering my eyes. I still wasn't used to this feeling of recognition for a job well done. When waiting tables my guests would always comment on my service and often wanted to tell the manager how well I took care of them, but recognition as a good *nurse* meant more to me, and made me feel I had finally arrived in the health care industry.

"We need more nurses like you!" Lucie said, smiling and looking around making sure everyone within earshot would hear.

"It truly was my pleasure—any time, Lucie!" I walked behind the desk to get the report from Tanya. I was grateful for Lucie's feedback, and more grateful that staff heard all of it—good press is important, especially for someone rebuilding a shattered life. What I thought was going to be a public hanging turned into my own miniature parade and it was a great start to my day. I hardly remembered helping Lucie the day before; I had to search my mind's whirlwind of memories from the previous shift for what *she* was recounting. I vaguely remembered taking her shoes off once she was in bed, and pressing on certain points of her feet a couple times since I still had my plastic gloves on. I wanted to use the gloves as much as possible before throwing them out since I was an environmentalist, and I believed in how much better someone could feel, even after a quick massage. I wanted to stay and revel in the feel-goods, but time was of the essence in this place and I had to use it wisely.

I had a couple good questions for Tanya, but I missed the majority of important ones. She was taken aback by the questions I asked, probably since the day before we had simply counted the narcotics and gone our separate ways. I asked about new orders and wound treatments but I could tell she wasn't as impressed as I wanted her to be. Being a new nurse was tough; sometimes faking it until you made it was all you could do. You could also work really hard and take care of your residents and most people would never worry about whether or not you had the knowledge a true nurse should possess. With that being said, I think about one of my favorite quotes. Helen Hayes said, "The expert in anything was once a beginner." Tanya left after our *thorough* report, slightly agitated, I sensed. I decided to start the med-pass a little earlier and gather supplies, and stock things on my cart that I would surely need. Glucometer strips and lancets for the diabetics, thermometer probes, gloves, wipes, juice, pudding and applesauce. I decided to make a list next time because surely I would miss something.

My med-pass started in the corner of the building, home to residents Jan Konkle and Leanne Donovan. It was a four-person room but currently only had two residents. I parked my cart in the tight corner and put the break on so it wouldn't roll away—I imagined it careening down the hills of San Francisco. I compared an out-of-control trolley to my haphazard med-pass. I started my rounds with great gusto and a positive outlook. Preparing Jan Konkle's medications was a journey in and of itself. She took seven different tablets which had to be crushed up very finely or else any bits she could feel with her tongue, she could spit out on your face, arms or scrubs. She also took two capsules that had to be poured into the applesauce. A nasal spray was also on her list of medications. That was a complete and utter joke. She was completely demented and entirely non-compliant. She was constantly yelling F bombs and other obscenities and always seemed like she was in a terrible mood. Some staff would joke about needing an exorcist to cure her… it was that bad unfortunately, and if this was sixty years in the past, an exorcist would definitely have been summoned… So if she took the spray, great. If not, I would still sign off on it as if she did. No one would ever know, and whether or not she took it wouldn't compromise her well-being or effect her care. In addition to that, she was a ward of the state, so no family would inquire about whether or not she is receiving her 17:00 nasal spray. I recall training one day with a seasoned nurse who recommended I didn't even try the nasal spray and to just sign for it. She also mentioned we should call the doctor and get it discontinued. I should have listened to her, but here's what happened: I gave Jan all her meds quite smoothly and came hopping back to the cart where the nurse was waiting. "I think she likes me, give me that nasal spray if you don't mind?" I accepted the challenge and was overly confident that Jan and I had developed a relationship.

"You sure? Nothing good gonna' happen, hero!" the nurse raised her eyebrows skeptically and laughed.

I foo-foo'd her and took the spray, hopping and bopping back in the room. Facing Jan, I told her slowly and loudly, "Jan! Here is your spray, okay? Breathe in through your nose on three!" I showed her the bottle and she looked at it and shook her head slightly. I lowered the bottle to her nose and just as I started to count she yelled, "AHH!" and slapped the bottle out of my hand to the opposite side of the room, "GET THE FUCK OUT! GET THE FUCK OUT!" she kept screaming the same four words at me until I left her bedside. I found the bottle under the empty bed across the room and as I picked it up, I looked to the doorway and found my orienting nurse and two CNAs watching and laughing hysterically. The nurse made eye contact with me and made an "I told you so!" with her face and eyes.

"Okay okay, shows over here! Nothing to see here!" I said in my best James Cagney voice, realizing that they were all from the Caribbean and probably didn't know who James Cagney was. I couldn't help but to laugh. Any time someone abruptly and viciously knocked something out of an unsuspecting person's hands, it was always funny. That same day they told everyone who visited our unit about the nasal spray air mail and everyone had a laugh. I would not ever be attempting to give Jan her nasal spray again. We would have to wait until we called the doctor for something else before asking about discontinuing it completely. If we had paged a doctor about a nasal spray they would have been furious.

Luckily, Jan was the first resident in the MAR, and the worst one. After her, it was all downhill from here… if downhill is a good thing. If it was a San Francisco downhill we'd be in trouble. The meds became less and less and the residents became more cooperative. Jan's roommate was not much better in terms of behavior, but a little more willing to take her crushed medicine in her applesauce. Leanne Donovan was a skinny, balding lady with multiple personality disorder. All her personalities were demented and rotten, but she was good at taking her medications in a timely fashion and with no persuasion needed. After every first bite, like clockwork, she would say in a loud, slow voice, "That-tastes-*terrible*!" And, every time I would say, "Oh, I know, don't worry it gets better!" And she would say while laughing, "I hope so!" She would then laugh some more and say something about her full name and something about the mystery as to who killed her father and who stole her baby. Some staff believed that all the things she was constantly muttering, must have actually happened to her, and maybe that was the reason for her psychosis. I had no idea whether it was true, but I felt bad for these two all the same. They'd both been in this corner room for the last ten years of their lives. A miserable way to spend the rest of their days and there was nothing you could do to make it any better for them.

I unlocked the brake and turned the cart ninety degrees up against the other wall, closer to the second corner room. I saw Jan's eyedrops on the cart that I'd forgotten to administer. I ran back in and said, "Hey Jan! Eye drops!" All of the sudden, she got quiet, inched up in her day chair, leaned back, looked at the ceiling and opened her eyes as wide as possible. Turns out, she loved her eyedrops! At least this return trip into the abyss was quick, easy and actually pleasant. I walked quickly out of the room before anything else could go wrong in this room of terror.

Up next was another quad corner room, with three residents in it. Wally, Jim, and Frank. I started Jim and Frank's meds first because Wally could wait till 17:00 exactly. His medications, Carbidopa/Levidopa, are Parkinson's medications, and need timely precision in administration. Nurses have to know how to organize their time, medications and supplies amid chaos and anarchy. If you fail at either of these skills, your shifts are longer and harder and chance for fatal errors increase.

Frank Dusen wore a beanie, glasses, three rosaries and dark and heavy clothes. He had a long and crooked nose that made Owen Wilson's look like a straight arrow. When he was hunched in his wheelchair roaming the halls, he looked like a fisherman muppet character and his appearance was quite comical. He only took four pills. He was my new favorite because of the small amount of attention he required. He took his pills whole and with ease. He only requested an Ensure if you didn't have one in hand already and I ruled that as reasonable.

Jim Moss was another easy resident. He lay in his bed all day long and never got up. He preferred it that way. He was able to transfer to wheel chairs with minimal assistance, but for some reason, refused to get out of bed each day. He answered simple questions with simple answers.

"Jim, you doing okay?" I asked, walking towards his bed.

"Yes I am" he shot back quickly as if his response had a time limit.

"…Good, good, going to the bathroom okay?" I was caught off guard but thought of another useful question as quickly as possible.

"Yes I am." He quipped back immediately.

Hmm, he's good at this, but I got another one on deck for you buddy! "That's excellent Jim! And are you in any pain today?"

"No pain" he said, glancing at me, then looking at his toes, as he did with every question.

Well I have a new favorite! Short and sweet. All the answers I want to hear. "Okay buddy, well that's good to hear. I have your medications here, are you ready?" I talked slower than normal, but I wonder if I'm insulting him because he hears and understands just fine.

"Okay," He opens his mouth waiting for the spoonful of applesauce and medication. He makes a loud, but concise "humm" sound as he eats it. The sound is similar to one a grandparent would make when pretending to playfully eat their grandchild's ear… it was very funny. I concluded that he must like eating. Even with his pureed diet of mush he ate every bite and made the same sound every time he swallowed the mashed up food.

On to Wally Lasiter, my friend with the Parkinson's. He looked like a tough guy. He was always in his chair, listening and/or watching TV with a word search forever incomplete on his bedside table. He was either word searching or coloring. Because of the Parkinson's his coloring was constantly outside the lines but I respected his efforts and his ability to accept imperfection. His mind was as sharp as a tack. I would soon find out that he memorized his daily blood pressures and could recall conversations from weeks before. Not bad for an 84 year old. I took a special liking to him because of the chief diagnosis of Parkinson's. My aunt was recently diagnosed and it was very sad to see. I made an impractical vow to always get his time-sensitive Carbidopa/Levadopa to him every day at 1700 on the dot. It was the least I could do. He also took an anti-hypotensive to prevent his BP from dipping too low. This was to counteract the anti-hypertensives he takes two times a day. Counterintuitive right? No it's not. Because the two drugs work on different receptors in the body, at least they do according to Dr. Menaja. Anyhow, I had to check his BP twice, once at 17:00 and once at 21:00. I hooked him up to the blood pressure cuff and started the machine. I still hadn't taken a manual blood pressure since I had started a couple of weeks earlier—modern day nursing, am I right?! Manual blood pressures were rarely used, unless the result was questioned for inaccuracy or the blood pressure instrument was not working on a resident, then we would break out the cuff and stethoscope and we'd look like real nurses! But I skipped all that every chance I got. While the BP was calculating I used the time to clear any hazards I saw or cleaned up the spilled food on the floor from lunch that was overlooked twelve different times by four different employees since noon. The first time I met Wally, he took his meds like a shot and it looked like he was trying to shake the remaining medications out of the cup and into his mouth. I almost said, "Stop shaking them, just dump them in your mouth." Then I recalled that Parkinson's caused tremors—I felt like an insensitive jerk and an even worse nurse. The truth is, in most long-term care facilities, you never had time to read all these charts and understand the condition, diagnosis, and background history of each resident. You knew the first or second diagnosis pertinent to the resident's care but after that, it might as well have been a guessing game.

The machine beeped, 90/56, HR 62. *Um, should I be worried? Probably not, right? Shit, I'm really out of my league here… The resident looks fine, shows no signs of hypotension, and states that he feels fine.* I got a brilliant idea. I returned to my medcart and checked all his recent blood pressures in the MAR—raw, hard data—nothing like numbers and statistics to draw conclusions and find answers. It appeared to be his range or baseline at this time every day, and this is why I needed to administer the anti-hypotensive Midodrine. As I walked back in to give him the last pill, I saw several cockroaches scurry away from the mountain of crumbs near Wally's bed. They saw me coming and took cover under the bed. I gave Wally the pill and would call housekeeping to sweep the floor. I wiped the sweat from my brow and finished him up.

"Good job, Wally; 94 over 56, heart rate 62," I told him as I turned to leave.

He raised his voice and stated in military fashion just like his roommate Jim Moss, "94 over 56. Heart rate 62!"

He looked at me the whole time as I stopped in my tracks to listen. *I am impressed, Wally!* I looked around, a bit confused. "Yes Sir! All clear on the western front, I'll see you after dinner, Sir! And drink some water to get your blood pressure back up!" He'd snapped me into a military mode I didn't know I had. After all, we did use military time, and the nursing discipline was much like the military. If you made mistakes they could be deadly, and you had to respect the clock and punctuality. *Maybe I could incorporate more military stuff into my daily routine?*

I returned to my cart to see one of the CNA's linen carts right behind it. The central supply man was making a last-minute inventory drop in our utility room as well, and his cart occupied the last bit of space that was free, so the corner was now very crowded. I maneuvered here and there with a half-turn and a hop between the linen cart, the boxes on the floor, and the supply cart, and freed my own cart enough to move one room down. I'd have to work on either timing or placement from now on, with these two rooms and the tight corner. One room further is where all the residents congregated—another roadblock. It was a minefield of linen carts, med-carts, wheelchaired residents, day chairs, broken beds, housekeeping carts, and plenty of other random big bulk objects taking up their half of the eight-foot-wide corridor. I had no difficulty steering my large cart, but keeping it stationary for parts of the med-pass seemed the best option.

Next up were Tabatha and Ruby, a very odd pair in a standard two-person room. Tabatha Patterson was a high-maintenance prissy, Tennessee native horse gal who was very particular about everything and let you know it. Apparently, she used to be a model which perhaps gave her a sense of entitlement or importance... she loved to mention this part of her life. She was Lucie Greer's best friend and the two were often found in each other's rooms or rolling up and down the hall together, to and from lunch and dinner. I gathered her medications and nasal spray and reintroduced myself, ready to give her the meds.

As soon as I put the cup in her hand, she looked from me to the cup and asked slowly, "What...are... these?"

Are you being funny, Tabatha? I was kind and resident but secretly, I felt agitated. "These are your five o'clock meds, Tabatha." (We didn't use military time with the residents because their heads might explode).

"Oh…" She looked at me and to the cup again, "What's… the… big… white… one?" She asked slowly.

"Potassium Chloride," I stated, growing imresident and keeping my responses short.

"Oh. What's… that… yellow… capsule?" She spoke even slower as if she was losing her breath.

"Omega-3 Fish oil." I exhaled and rolled my eyes. She couldn't see my eye roll because she was getting ready for the next question, looking in the cup.

"Oh…how… about… that… circular… one?" she asked, glancing from me to the cup and back again.

"Pepcid, and the last one is Florastor, to help regulate your bowels," I said louder as if to embarrass her in front of her roommate in the bed next to her, but who wasn't *really* there. I immediately felt guilty.

"Oh! I know that one!" she said irritated, loudly, and quite faster than all the other words she'd just spoken.

Oh my lord; Tabatha! Maybe she did actually know that one. Who cares. On to the next one—her roommate, Ruby.

Ruby had her bed against the wall with a floor mattress next to it and full bed rails up because she was a fall risk. Ruby's mind was completely gone, so it was difficult to get her to take her meds, but otherwise, she was an easy resident. I just had to be vigilant so she wouldn't fall and break her hip or head. She took her medicine crushed with applesauce and nothing else. She was German and often went from English to German and back again. Sometimes she would speak only German for days at a time. Occasionally she would clench her teeth and jaw and refuse medication. You had the choice of documenting it as a refusal or coming back in fifteen minutes and trying again. If you came back, you would have to store the medication somewhere, keep track of it, and come back quickly, otherwise, you could forget about it and by the time you found it at 2300 (11:00 p.m.), it would be too late to legally give it, plus the resident would most likely be sleeping. Ruby liked singing. It was more of a hum. No words. Just a tune. One tune. "Silent Night." Yes. It was Christmas time all year round in Ruby's head. She actually had a beautiful voice, much like an opera singer and everyone loved listening to her, staff included. She took my medication this time, thank goodness! I could move on. I was running behind so I quickly got back to my cart, unlocked the wheel, and pushed and tried to recall details of the next residents. I didn't remember much.

Leslie Dawson and Barbara Watkins shared a standard double. They were both fall risks so they had their beds to the wall with floor mattresses (so much more room for activities). They both had severe dementia as well, but were fan favorites of all the staff. They were perhaps the most challenging residents on my unit. Leslie Dawson loved to get up and try to walk. She'd take two or three unsteady steps and find a wall or door knob, lowering herself down to the floor; if she didn't outright fall. All fall-risk residents had bed alarms that would beep very loudly and could be heard a hundred yards down a hallway. The problem was that you could be that hundred yards down the hall and by the time you sprinted and found the alarm, the resident could be on the floor. Vigilant eyes and constant room checks were the only way to truly prevent falls. Leslie refused her meds and didn't believe that I was a nurse—she thought I was an old boyfriend trying to trick her. I stayed and tried to reason with her, but after five minutes and no progress, I moved on to Barbara. Barbara was also a fall risk but somewhere in her warped mind, she knew her feet couldn't handle the weight of her body. She was still likely to roll out of bed daily. She was also a diabetic so I needed to check her sugar and administer insulin before the food trays arrived. I had four other diabetics I needed to get to. Barbara was completely compliant and absolutely delightful. She spoke in a slurred, high-pitched voice. Her favorite word was *"Aight"* and she always said it with enthusiasm. Giving out all these pills was a boring, tedious task and anyone could do it. Nursing skills such as injections made me feel like a real nurse doing something important. I remember to a tee, the exact order, and process, of drawing and administering insulin, from nursing school six years before. I told Barbara what I was going to do, and I did it. She smiled a wide, toothless smile and said, "Aight!" I thanked her and went on to the next one.

Next up was my news correspondent, Lucie Greer, and her sidekick Julie Walton. They shared a double room and Lucie was the *big sister* who always looked out for Julie from the confines of her bed. She made sure Julie ate and that the staff was taking good care of her. In between caring for Julie from afar, she always watched the news and repeated everything that the CNN anchors would say to anyone who would listen. Completely compliant and very pleasant, I could do her medications in less than thirty seconds. She warned me of a virus called Corona something or another and I paid her no mind. There was always some type of virus coming out of some corner of the world that everyone would freak out about. SARS, swine flu, bird flu, mad cow disease. I wasn't too worried and countered with some type of "Oh yeah?" or "Hm. Very interesting." I gave her her two meds and went on to her roommate. Julie was hemiplegic (total one-sided weakness) from a stroke or CVA, so she was another bed-to-the-wall resident, with a floor mattress and side rails. She was also very pleasant. No matter what you did or what you said, Julie would smile ear to ear and say, "Oh... yeah..." in a very calm, quiet voice. I guess she was happy to have the company, no matter how fleeting, inattentive or invasive it was. She would light up when she saw me and that made me happy—I chose to believe her happiness was specific to me. Lucie told me about Julie and how she loved her gin and tonics. I wondered if her drinking was what lead to the hypertension (high blood pressure) that had caused the CVA (cerebrovascular accident) and if maybe I would have shared the same fate if I had continued on my booze-filled path. Julie always had a buildup of gunk and eye boogers in both eyes. For some strange reason, I really enjoyed cleaning it all out. I would douse both eyes with her prescribed lubricating eye drops. Then I'd take a tissue for each eye and carefully wipe from the inner canthus (corner) and out, like they taught me in nursing school. I enjoyed helping residents directly and immediately. Looking at the finished result was extremely satisfying to me. Sometimes, she would squeeze her eyes shut (still smiling) and I would have to carefully pry them open. I loved a challenge, and not too many things came easy around here. I was used to the obstacles and problems guaranteed to arise. On to the next one!

Moving along, I unlocked my cart and swung it almost irresponsibly, ten feet down to the next room where Britt Carter awaited my visit. He occupied a single room (lucky!) but contrary to the solitary lifestyle he paid for, he had many visitors all day long. I found Jeffrey Pratt standing next to his bed talking about the dinner trays that were due to arrive any minute. *Should I kick him out?* I decided to let him stay and asked Britt my standard array of questions. He answered quickly, without even acknowledging my physical presence, and continued his conversation with Jeffrey as I took his blood pressure. I positioned the machine so I could see it from the doorway while I gathered his medications. I had all seven pills he needed, except for the midodrine, which was contingent on his BP results. The machine beeped and read 90/48, HR 60. *A record low! Congratulations Britt, lets see what you've won! Well it's ten milligrams of Midodrine to keep the blood pressure from going any lowerrrr!* Because of my experience with Wally, I remembered to check the MAR to make sure his blood pressure was within his baseline range, and it was. I popped the Midodrine through the foil and in the medication cup and brought him his whole pills. I placed it on the bedside table and stood between the two men, waiting for Britt to take the meds. After a couple of seconds they both looked at me, as if to say, "Okay nurse, what are you still doing here?" *Should I stay or should I go now?* the song by the Ramones rang in my head. Nursing 101 required me to stay and watch the resident take the medicine… While I was dancing around in my head, I heard Britt say in a deep voice, "I'll take them, don't worry." He rolled his eyes towards Jeffrey, and Jeffrey laughed a bit.

Embarrassed, I turned and walk out, saying cheerfully, "Okay, don't forget about them!" *I hope I didn't insult him…* "And drink some water! Your blood pressure is too low." I got no response from either of them. I would have to check back to make sure he kept his word and that his blood pressure didn't fall any lower. In the meantime, on to the next one.

I pulled my cart down to the next room, another single. Jordan Cliff. Apparently, Jordan used to be a pimp in Alabama. He had a small afro and was a big boy. He also had hemiplegia from a stroke that affected the right side of his body. He was a diabetic, and also had hypertension. He didn't speak much, but when he did, you had to concentrate very hard and use context to figure out what he was saying. It was garbled like a staticky radio, or as if he had the proverbial and eternal marbles in his mouth. The only phrase Jordan said that was always and absolutely crystal clear was, "I DON'T GIVE A FUCK!" He said this when he didn't want to take medications or was being non-compliant with regard to something else. He took his crushed medication in chocolate pudding and only chocolate pudding. I remembered this from the day before. He made me redo all his meds when I presented them in applesauce. You can imagine the anger I felt when he refused to take the medicine that had taken me ten minutes to prepare. So this time, I made sure I had chocolate pudding for this diva.

I heard the food tray arrive at the corner. I rushed back into Jordan's room and take his blood sugar. It was 358. I had to check the MAR and see what his sliding scale called for. The sliding scale will tell you how many units of fast-acting insulin the resident gets, depending on his blood sugar result. 358 called for ten units. *Congratulations Jordan Cliff! Well, it's ten units of Humalog insulin! Injected subcutaneously, this injection will lower your blood sugar almost immediately and prevent you from going into diabetic ketoacidoooo-sis!* I drew it up, walked back into the room, and asked him where he wanted the needle. He lifted up his shirt, looking unsure if he really wanted me to stick him with the instrument of torture. *Relax Jordan, it's not that bad, especially for a tough pimp like you.* I grabbed some belly fat and stuck it in at a forty-five-degree angle, and I started singing *"Pimps don't cryyy, no they don't shed a tearrrr!"* He laughed at the Eva Mendez song I sang to him. He liked to be called a pimp and when you asked him, he confirmed that he really used to pimp women. I laughed out loud and patted him on the back. He was really likable, especially after laughing at my jokes. Our moment over, I moved on. Still two more diabetics to get to before the dinner trays got to them.

I walked out to see the trays hadn't moved. *What the fuck!* I walked into the resident lounge, where all the loafers sat and hung out when they weren't working. They weren't even on a break, just not working. I found all three of my CNAs sitting in the lounge. One of them looked like she was sleeping. I poked my head in and said, "Dinner's here." Two of them looked up but none of them acknowledged me with words. I walked back out, knowing they heard me, but convinced they weren't moving fast enough. Food was the only thing the residents looked forward to. That and maybe Jeopardy or Family Feud, or a daily recreation activity in the large dining hall in the center of the building. I knew what it was like to have food be the only thing to look forward to. I spent two months in county jail after my second DWI. In jail, there is nothing to do but work out and eat, and I'd be damned if these elderly people were getting cold food when everyone in jail enjoyed their meals in a hot and timely fashion. I let this one slide but paid close attention to when the CNAs came back out. I couldn't start too many fires with the staff this early in my career. If I got into it with too many CNAs so soon, I'd lose any respect and admiration before I'd even gained it. Professor Ruffini warned of CNAs and their work ethics—or lack thereof. I didn't really believe it, but what did I know? *Absolutely nothing.* It took close to ten minutes before all three CNAs were up and at 'em. The trays began to make it to their final destinations.... at a rate slower than molasses in Alaska. Dinner trays were another thing I would have to remedy, but first I needed to perfect my craft —especially my sluggish med-pass. There were plenty of starfish here that needed saving, but I could barely walk through the sand yet.

Next up was Corey Chapman. He was one of three in a quadruple corner room. He was sixty years old and morbidly obese. I estimated 400 pounds. I could have checked his chart for that information but nobody had time for that. Corey was always grumpy and angry. He always complained about someone or something. As soon as you left his presence, you would be the subject of his complaints. I felt for him, just like I felt for all these residents. I wouldn't be the happiest person either if I was stuck in this geriatric prison. Corey continued to talk and move while I took his BP, which could upset the mechanisms of the machine and call for a repeat blood pressure. I asked him politely to try and stay still and be quiet. "Okay, okay," he practically shouted at me. I took a deep breath and went to empty his urinal. He decided he needed to instruct me on how to do this. Elderly people love giving direction to younger folks when performing simple tasks—like dumping urine in a toilet and flushing. I entertained his need for participation and did every little thing the way he asked. These instructions did not help the BP machine but it performed its function even with all the movement and yelling from its subject. I dished out Corey's medications and waited while he took them. Once the medications were on his table, he stopped talking and focused on taking them. *Well that's one thing you got going for you buddy!* He swallowed them all and told me what the day shift CNA did or said. I turned and walked out, trying not to listen. "I have to go, Corey; we'll catch up later, okay?" I promised emptily as I left. I knew he'd find some other victim to listen to his rants.

"Okay, okay," he shouted as I walked away to my med-cart.

His roommate was another Parkinson's resident who was completely bed-ridden. I realized that his 1700 carbidopa/levodopa was now forty minutes late and that I'd have to make a promise to him as well about the punctuality of his medications. He also got eye drops, a blood pressure check, and a quick wipe down from me. I administered his crushed medication in apple sauce and looked for the third and final resident in the quadruple room.

The resident was nowhere to be found. Dillan Schmidt. He was a double leg amputee with bilateral (both sides) prostheses. He was the one racing up and down the halls with the walker. When I first saw him, I had no idea he was working with all the hardware below both thighs. He also had permission to go to the corner store for anyone and everyone. It was probably about a fifth of a mile away. He made this trip about seven times a day. He would pick up coffee for staff, snacks, sandwiches and sodas for residents, but he would do it for a fee. He never worked out a price or percentage but people tipped him and this was his secondary income in addition to his social security. It gave him plenty of exercise and more importantly, a purpose. Anyhow, he couldn't be found so I skipped his multi-vitamin and calcium supplement. He could wait.

Next up was Agatha Monroe who was the only occupant in a double room. The bed next to hers was full of books, magazines, and newspapers. Her two large wardrobes had more newspapers and magazines on top of each one. I didn't want to imagine what was inside those wardrobes. She wasn't blind, but her eyes always looked shut. She was another diabetic, and the food tray was right outside her room. I quickly informed her who I was, and what I was about to do. Her sugar was 130. *Thank god. No insulin.* Although I enjoyed giving injections and felt like a real nurse when doing so, I was still behind so this time-saver was a blessing. I got her medications. Turns out she didn't get sliding scale insulin but she did have a standing dose of eight units before dinner—I still had to give her an injection after all. I got the syringe, and found her insulin among the nine other vials of insulin. There was fast-acting and long-lasting insulin. I multiplied the two types of insulin by four residents plus extra vials from expired or discharged residents plus expired insulin we could no longer give and found out that's why half the top drawer was full of insulin. When administering insulin, you had to check the vial you were drawing from multiple times before administering it. If you gave twenty units of a fast-acting insulin when you were supposed to give the long-lasting, it could kill the resident, especially if they were a labile diabetic with a low blood sugar already.

"Here is your insulin, Agatha," I said loudly, because she was hard of hearing.

"Right arm, please," she said, lifting up her sleeve with her left hand.

"On three; okay?!"

"Mm-hm," she nodded, closing her eyes even more.

"One…" and before I even got to two—BOOM! I stuck her with the needle. A little trick I learned from an orthopedic surgeon in the ER—he'd used the same trick while snapping a middle finger back in place. The middle finger had looked like an uppercase L. I liked this trick. The resident had waited for the three count but before the surgeon even got to the number two, the finger was back in place. Ann didn't seem to mind my dishonest counting trick. She was used to getting stuck with needles a dozen times a day.

I gave her her eyedrops, which she did herself and she asked for tissues before her self-administration—which I had forgotten. I gave her her nasal spray, which she did herself, and all the pills and capsules of medicine she would dump in her mouth all at once. Through her barely-opened eyelids, she examined the medicine. Her ninety-two-year-old eyes could discern that I had missed one of her pills.

"It looks like I'm missing the magnesium oxide," she said glumly.

"Okay let me take a look at that," I said as I took the med cup and went back to the room. *How the hell…?* I had to restart at her section of the MAR and go medication by medication and compare it to the bingo cards to find out which pills I'd already popped and confirmed that I did in fact miss the magnesium oxide. After another five minutes—which seemed like an eternity—I went back into the room and gave her the medicine cup. "You were right! I missed the mag-ox!" I can admit when I'm wrong. I have no pride or ego, or at least not as much as I used to, thanks to my Alcohol Support Groups. She mumbled and said, "Hmm," and that was that.

By this time, all the trays were out and most of the residents were eating. I banged out the next two residents, who were fairly simple. The one after them was another diabetic and I realized this guy had already finished eating and I hadn't checked his blood sugar! Diabetic keto-acidosis here we come. *Shit! What do I do?!* The point of getting blood sugar results before meals was to treat the existing blood sugar before the resident ate and brought more carbohydrates in. I would later learn that pre-meal blood sugars were missed frequently. Normally it wasn't a problem, but if a resident was a labile—or sensitive—diabetic, they could crash if you gave them too much. I was still out of my league here. Nursing school hadn't prepared me for missed blood sugars and insulin. I could text a nurse from my family or one of my nurse friends or ask another nurse down the hall, or Google it. I decided it wasn't enough of a big deal to consult an off-duty nurse from my network. I chose Google and found nothing useful or clear, only advertisements for glucometer instruments and discounts on insulin prescriptions. I decided to improvise and 'fake it until I make it.' Kellan Quinn's blood sugar was 356! It couldn't have been because of the food he just ate?! I looked at his sliding scale and he got ten units. If it was above 400 it would have been a real issue because I would have had to call the doctor. I gave him his ten units and made sure I checked him as soon as 21:00 (9:00 p.m.) came around. I wrote myself a note. Because of my ADHD and the fact that I couldn't take my Adderall because of the Board of Nursing program and its drug testing, I had to write everything down because I could be forgetful. I realized now that I had to heavily rely on this note-taking—people's lives were at stake… kind of. There were a couple of other loose ends I had to finish up, but I was done with the med-pass at 1830 since I had decided to start earlier this day. I pushed my cart the forty yards back to the nursing desk, where I sat down, flustered, and exhaled loudly. I thought no one was around, but Jeffrey Pratt was sitting on the other side near the corner where the utility room was located. He was hidden behind half a dozen fat charts lined on the half-wall above the desk. He could often be found there. He slid back into my field of vision.

"You all right bro?" he asked while staring intently down the hall. He looked like he was waiting for something to jump out so he could wrangle it. He was 6'2" and a heavy man. He talked loudly and disregarded his personal hygiene.

"Yeah just fine man, thanks for asking," I scoffed. "Just gotta give my feet a rest."

"Yeah man, don't get burnt out, all these new nurses come in, do a month of this shit, and then decide they can't do it anymore, or it's not worth it," he said wisely.

"Really?" The thought of burning out had never occurred to me. I was a young buck with infinite patience and a whole lot of debt. Burning out was not an option.

"Oh yeah, the amount of work this place makes these nurses do, it's no wonder. Just take it easy and don't overwork yourself."

Wow! What sage advice, Jeff! Is this what you tell these damn CNAs? If the CNAs were following Joeffrey's' orders, then the mystery as to why they were so lazy and slow was solved. I smiled and nodded, thanking him. I could see him being an ally in the future. He wasn't a resident of mine, but he was another one who was always around the whole building, visiting all the other residents. He could be found outside smoking a lot of the time, too. The first time I saw him he was wheeling another resident to the lobby and I wondered if he was a volunteer, visitor or employee. He wasn't dressed like an employee so I figured visitor or volunteer.

I got up five minutes later and found him in the kitchenette across from the nursing desk preparing a basin full of six ice waters for six lucky winners. Would you look at that! Our best CNA was a resident!

Dinner was over and the kitchen staff returned to take the six-foot food carts back to the dungeon where the kitchen was. I saw Jeffrey Pratt hustling in and out of all the rooms, returning the half-eaten trays to the food cart. He really was doing a lot of CNA work. I felt bad that he was doing this. No one made him do it, and he wasn't getting paid for it, either. He enjoyed helping others and I supposed this was *his* purpose. He would do great in my Alcohol Support Groups—helping others was the way to stay sober. I marveled at Jeoffrey's spirit and energy and thought that maybe these things he did keep him truly happy. I had plenty of my own work to do so I let Jeffrey do his thing. I stayed seated as I looked through and signed the TAR while I continued to let my legs rest. Documentation and desk work would be good friends of mine because they allowed my feet some time off. Standing on your feet in one position for more than fifteen minutes could really take its toll, as I would soon find out. I thought about the collective 2.5 miles I would have to ride to get back home. As I signed the TAR, I saw dozens of blank spaces where nurses did not sign. I would never be one of those nurses. I finished signing the TAR and flagged several treatments that I could finish up now, and some of them that would have to be done later because they had only been done three-and-a-half hours earlier by the 7 to 3 nurse. One of them belonged to Adrian Larson.

Adrian apparently had been homeless somewhere in New England one winter, and had fallen asleep in an abandoned motel. He'd woken up with severe frost bite. How he came to New Jersey I'm not sure; I think it had something to do with his sister living in the area. Adrian had many diagnoses, was on several narcotics for pain, was severely cognitively impaired, and in addition to all this, had an unstageable pressure wound with tunneling. Tunneling is exactly what it sounds like, it was a deep crater in his buttocks that also went laterally under the skin, like a tunnel off to the side of what could be seen. I would describe him as *rotting away in bed* because that was the most accurate description. It was very sad to see, but this taught me a lesson about nurses and good nurses. A nurse would approach him and set out to do the treatment, only to retreat and leave after Adrian merely said the word, "No." When the resident said no, the nurse could document the treatment as a refusal. Nurses could not force the resident to do anything, so many got away without doing the treatment, which is why the wound kept worsening. The good nurse would stay there and debate and try and persuade him to allow them to perform this vital treatment (if the good nurse had time and patience after a grueling first half med-pass). With enough gumption and perseverance, the nurse would get their way. A second pair of hands was always helpful but usually never to be found. His treatment required removing the old bandages, cleaning the wound with normal saline and gauze, patting the exposed tissue dry, then packing the crater with medication-saturated gauze, then applying a large bandage over everything and taping the bandage to the skin. Since it was his right buttocks, you would have to lift the buttocks up and apply the adhesive tape, and then let the right buttocks fall so you knew it was applied adequately; otherwise, it would just come off the first time he moved in bed. I dreaded my wound date with Adrian but tried to think positively about the experience I would gain by treating his enormous wound. I had done some other minor treatments—nystatin powder in various skin folds of various residents. Lotion on various limbs of various residents.

I ate a quick dinner and drank a ton of water while at the desk. I was fed, hydrated, rested, and right on track. All my treatments were done except for Adrian's, and I could start my 21:00 med-pass an hour in advance to ensure most residents got their medicine at a reasonable time, and they could go to bed early. I checked blood pressures and blood sugars, put residents in their beds, tucked them in, and turned out the lights. Mr. Potter's blood sugar came down to 157. He would require two units of short-acting insulin according to his sliding scale, on top of his forty-eight units of long-lasting insulin. I generally questioned a lot of stuff, even when I had no business doing so, but as his sugar had been so high earlier, I gave the insulin that was ordered and didn't think twice about it. I figured the MDs knew that he liked snacking and liked sugar and that's why he had all this insulin coming in. I muttered something about laying off the sweets but Mr. Potter was very forgetful so I figured I'd best leave it be. My Alcohol Support meetings taught me not to get involved in other people's business, just to follow the rules and keep my side of the street clean; but what about when I was the nurse responsible for residents who couldn't care for themselves? Was I being judgmental when trying to teach residents to not eat sugar? Was I not minding my own business? It's a fine line to walk when caring for others who may not know what is best for themselves. Either way, it was time to move; Adrian would be waiting.

I parked my cart at the nursing station and then went around the corner to open the treatment cart. It had similar dimensions to the medication cart but was about half the size. It was filled with gauze, ointments, cotton balls, saline, popsicle sticks, bandages, ace bandages, ice packs, warm packs, and much more. I found all the supplies I needed and lay them out on the top surface of the cart. I peeled open the bandage, pulled it out, and wrote my initials, the date, and the time. I put it back in the package. I pulled out some gauze, soaked it with normal saline, and put it on top of the bandage. I brought out double the amount of gauze and put it on top of the wet gauze. I wore two gloves on each hand which is technically a big "no-no" according to the standard nursing procedures but was so practical, that it's hard not to indulge once in a while. I would be removing the top set of gloves after cleaning the wound, revealing fresh clean ones to add the new medication and gauze, while staying with the same resident, so this further justified my rule-breaking (I wouldn't be bringing any of his germs to other residents). I scooped up all my supplies and headed into the room.

"Hey Adrian, time to do your wound, buddy!" I said enthusiastically and sternly all at the same time. I was greeted with a:

"Fuck you, you mother fucker!" he yelled while looking at me. He glanced at the supplies, then back to me. "What is all that fucking shit?!" His face reddened, frightened and uncertain.

"These are some cleaning supplies to help that wound on your butt!" *Cleaning supplies? I sounded like a janitor.*

"Fuck that, you fucking fuck, I don't want them," he spoke loudly but a little calmer. He looked away as if ignoring me would make me leave sooner. He must have been in the habit of getting his way with little resistance. Lucky for him *and* his wound, I had infinite patience and a new outlook on life, since getting sober. It was God's will—and maybe a doctor's order that I clean and dress his wound. I took a deep breath, put the supplies down on the bedside table, and got close to his bed. I wondered what I would say and if it would convince him. I remembered Tanya saying how Tylenol before treatments was always a good idea, and that Adrian especially liked his Tylenol. I remembered he had an order for Tylenol, 'Q 6 hours PRN' (the Q stood for every, and the PRN meant as needed—every six hours as needed) and knew that since it was 2200 already and I hadn't given him any Tylenol, he could have some.

"Adrian," I said in a low calm voice, "I'm going to get you Tylenol and I'm going to come back and we'll do this wound together. We have to do it so you can get better. Sound like a plan?"

He thought about it for a second, looked at his TV, and said, "Fine." He surrendered easily and I was pumped with this easy concession! After this win, I supposed the other nurses hadn't been trying too hard. I pranced and danced out of the room and got to the med-cart and opened it—except it wouldn't open because I had locked it. I looked to the treatment cart for the key; surely they were there. Beads of sweat ran down my forehead; I literally felt my armpits sweating. I started to panic and looked all around the desk, lifting papers up, looking on the floor. No one was around to help—or to criticize. *Damn!* My head was spinning with fear and my absent ego was now resurfacing and swelling. I worried about my appearance before worrying about my residents; and how I was locked out of the carts which held everything they needed. *Am I going to be known as the nurse who lost the keys on his second day? How will I look to my peers and supervisors?!* I took a moment to think. I started to retrace my steps—*Thanks, mom. Thanks, Grandma.* I was always losing shit my whole life—the doctors blamed the ADHD—and retracing my steps was always the first advice I heard. I walked back into Adrian's room and there they were, next to his messy dinner tray that no one had cleared. The relief I felt may have been the best feeling of my life. Phew! It was a good day, but unfortunately, this wouldn't be the last time I panicked over misplaced keys. I was relieved but projected my frustration into and onto the person that was supposed to clear this tray and didn't. No time to digress. I ran back out to the med-cart and got the Tylenol, ripped open the MAR, found his section, found the separate PRN page, and signed the date, time, initials, and result. I prematurely signed that the result was an effective one…with a 'plus' sign. I ran back to the room after a deep breath and acted calm and poised in front of Adrian.

"Here's the Tylenol, my friend." I handed him the medicine cup and gave him the ice water Jeffrey Pratt had brought hours earlier. By now it had little ice but was still refreshing and would do the trick to get the Tylenol down. He threw it back like a shot of whiskey and found the straw with his mouth, closed one eye, and sucked intensely on the straw. With his open eye, he stared me down, making sure I was making no sudden moves. He lowered the head of the bed all by himself, and I couldn't help but think that he knew this routine and that maybe certain nurses had a pretty high batting average when it came to treating his wound. He even turned by himself and grabbed the opposite bed rail! Talk about prejudging someone— Adrian was totally compliant and somewhat competent when it came to participating in his care, once he actually agreed to participate! I quickly took off the brief (diaper) to get to the massive abyss in the man's buttocks. The bandage and the four feet of rolled gauze were completely saturated with blood. I forgot to make note of what the initials, date, and time were, on the bandage I pulled off. I estimated that no one had changed this bandage for at least forty-eight hours, but what did I know. I had all the blood-drenched bandages and gauze in both my hands. *Fuck! The trash can! What would I do with this massive heap of biohazard in my hands?!* The lack of preparation haunted me. I had gotten all the supplies but had failed to consider an exit strategy! Adrian looked strong enough to hold on for a couple more minutes, so I ran to the trash and threw it all out, then pushed the trash back with my foot to the side of the bed where I was stationed. I took the saline-saturated gauze and began to blot and dab the cave that was this man's rump. I made note that the flesh was red and no odor could be detected. This was a good sign. After what I believed to be a thorough cleaning, I decided it was time to start patting dry the flesh. My game plan was interrupted by my angry customer.

"Come on, come on!" Adrian said almost politely, but imresidently all the same. He got louder, "COME ON COME ON YOU FUCK!" Adrian lost any patience he'd mustered a few minutes earlier.

I sweat even harder. "Okay buddy, we're almost done, give me one more minute!" I responded ever so kindly given the circumstances, surprising myself. He replied with an easy, calm, "Okay."

What the hell?! This guy is so hot and cold! Then I remembered one of his psych diagnoses was bipolar disorder. Could this be a manifestation? Either way, I took the top gloves off to get to the clean new gloves underneath them. I took the medication and doused the ball of gauze that would call this gluteal cavern home for the next sixteen hours. I packed it to the side where the tunnel started and wondered how far left it went.... I took the extra long Q-Tip that I'd brought just in case and started to poke around. It finally hit "bottom" and I could estimate the depth of the tunneling. Thank God! I put some more medication saturated gauze behind it. The wound was now full of the medication-saturated gauze. I put the time-stamped bandage on top and taped it to his skin, holding up the right butt cheek and then letting it fall. I exhaled and told Adrian he could roll onto his back and raise the head of the bed up once more. I secured his brief and replaced his gown over his pelvic area. My lower back was burning; I'd been bent over this whole time. Nursing 101, raise the bed to working height—more missed preparation. I'd try not to make that mistake again! Overall I felt great because I was triumphant in this episode of Adrian and the cave. I thanked Adrian and he said, "Yeah, okay." I ditched my gloves, cleaned up the bedside table, washed my hands, and got the hell out of Dodge! As I walked out Adrian said, "Hey! Wait!"

I stopped in my tracks hoping for and expecting a grateful "Thank you," but that was wishful thinking. "Yes, buddy. What's up? What do you need?" I stepped backward a couple of paces so we could see each other.

He paused and looked at me. "FUCK YOU, YOU FUCK!" he screamed, while maintaining eye contact, and then turned his attention back to the TV. As I returned to the nursing station I was grateful I didn't take his comments personally. I sat down, and exhaled a long exasperated breath. It felt good helping this man, but damn did I work for it! I recalled one of my brother's favorite quotes, "Without a dull and determined effort, there can be no great and glorious achievement." I laughed, thinking about the ending of our joint escapade.

As soon as I caught my breath, Jeffrey Pratt was at the side of the nursing station leaning over, practically spitting in my face. I wheeled my computer chair back a couple of feet to evade the barrage of saliva. He yelled about some "loafers" which was confusing to me. I didn't know if he meant shoes, bread, or something else. He was talking about the CNAs whose work he did on the regular. I entertained his rant and tried to make myself busy. He took the hint and went about his nightly rounds to all his customers and audiences.

The rest of the night was uneventful. I straightened up the desk, put charts back in their proper place, and finished some other paperwork. I looked around for any charts that might have been flagged with new doctor's orders that I'd need to carry out before leaving; there were none, thankfully. The overnight nurse from the staffing agency arrived late, but I gave a decent report all the same. I thought about the previous night with Rita and the useful information that the incoming nurse needed. She didn't seem that interested, probably since this was a temporary post for her. We counted drugs and I got the hell out of there. My job was rewarding but excruciatingly exhausting.

I got on my bike and started the first leg of my journey—a mile-long bike ride to the train station. Then I waited fifteen minutes for the 12:07 back to the city where I lived. The train ride, the second leg of my commute, was six minutes. The train was full of folks coming back from New York City. They all had headphones on or were talking on the phone. A seemingly homeless lady walked up and down with her cart, asking for money. I gave her a loose dollar bill from my back scrub pocket. I got to my hometown train station. From there I biked another 1.5 miles to my apartment. I locked my bike up in the back of the *father and son* dentist's office. During my commute home I remembered things I'd forgotten to do but was lucky because none of the forgotten tasks warranted a phone call to the unit. I got home at 12:30 and immediately threw my clothes in the dirty laundry hamper and showered. I didn't need any piss, shit, blood, or any other bodily fluid getting all over my apartment. I brushed my teeth in the shower to save time. I wanted to sit and watch TV but I was way too tired for that. I said the prayers that my Alcohol Support Group taught me and fell right to sleep next to my girlfriend, Candace.

Chapter 3

February 19th

Gratitude lists

After sleeping for nearly nine hours, I woke up at 10 a.m. I swung my feet to the side of the bed. Before I get up, I say my arsenal of prayers which include the Serenity Prayer, the Lord's Prayer, and several prayers I learned at my Alcohol Support Groups—about helping others, deflating your ego, and asking for sobriety, strength, and patience throughout the day. I let my feet dangle over the bed and as I started to put weight on them, my heels screamed with the pain of pins and needles. Standing on your feet all day sucks, and your feet and heels are the biggest victims, feeling it the most.

I got to my living room and began my daily routines and rituals. Since Candace was at work, my routines and rituals were mine, and mine alone. I turned on my Spotify playlist and played it through the Bluetooth speaker—my gym playlist to get me pumped up for the day. I cooked some quick eggs and ate some peanut butter toast. Since I woke up later than usual I was only able to have a quick workout before going straight to my 12:15 Alcohol Support Group downtown. I took my bike to the gym, locked it up in the lobby, worked out, then biked to the meeting a couple of blocks away where I carried my bike down to the church basement so as not to tempt any bike thieves. At the meeting, I got my daily dose of spirituality and fellowship and then biked back to my apartment. I biked everywhere. It was my main mode of transportation because the DMV took my license for ten years, after my third DWI. If I ever mentioned how the DMV took my license at an Alcohol Support Group meeting, a wise and sober alcoholic might say that no one took it from me, but rather I forfeited it because of my reckless and selfish behavior, and I could never disagree with those sage old drunks. Alcohol Support Groups focused on changing behavior and especially the thinking and thought processes that led to misconduct and misbehavior. The groups taught you new ways to think and focused on seeing life and situations from different perspectives. Without this type of support and newfound consideration, I would have been dead or back in jail… I'm sure of it. I lived for these meetings and the clarity they provided my distorted psyche.

I avoided Uber and Lyft altogether. The rides were expensive and unreliable. If a trip was too long by bike I would bite the bullet and pay for one of these rideshare services. Even during the winter, I rode my bike everywhere—I just prepared for it. I'd wear a long sleeve shirt under a heavy Goldfang sweatshirt hoodie with a matching Goldfang winter hat to match. I'd wear two pairs of gloves—one, a thin skin-tight glove made for dexterity, and the next, a heavier mitten/glove combo made for skiing. Your hands get the coldest on a bike during the northeast winters. They took the brunt of the cold air you'd be working against. I wore long johns under heavy gray sweat pants. I'd wear my trusty sunglasses. I wore two pairs of socks and regular running sneakers. My bike was a Trek hybrid.

On the way to the gym, I passed through blocks and blocks of Spanish neighborhoods. I listened to a lot of salsa, bachata, and some banda and always wondered if I would be welcome at their summer barbecues because of our similar taste in music. Although it was mainly Spanish in this area, many of the houses on the main street were converted into doctor's offices, law offices, offices for tax advisors, accounting services, and so on. I was in the right lane of the four-way highway, hoping I wouldn't get hit by a drunk driver. *Wouldn't that be ironic.* "Habitual drunk driver killed by drunk driver" would be the headline. It was early enough in the day that drunk drivers were few and far between so I decided not to worry too much. I saw the 227 bus going the other way. I had a monthly pass so I knew all the drivers and recognized Cesar driving it. I saluted him, and he honked his horn in response.

I got to the gym at 11:00 a.m. and wasted no time getting right into it. I waved, acknowledging all the other everyday gym rats. We rarely talked—just the way I liked it. This was my time; my workout lasted close to an hour and I was on my way out the door, sweating. Since I had limited time I had tried to do all my different exercises back to back and with little breaks.

I rode the two blocks to the Episcopalian church that was gracious enough to host us every Thursday at noon. I saw Lonnie and Fred sitting outside, greeting incoming alcoholics and addicts. This meeting was always interesting, although most meetings did have their unique flair and flavor. This one was particularly interesting because aside from our core group of regulars, we would have big finance guys, pharmaceutical people, and all other types of businessmen and women in town in need of a lunch break meeting. We met people from all over the East Coast and Midwest, and sometimes others from the West Coast and if we were really lucky, Europe or Asia. No matter where you were in the world, the alcoholic support groups were there to be found and their message was always the same. We had some southies in from Boston who told us funny stories but managed to get everyone teary-eyed at the end of their anecdotes. I always admired storytellers who could make you laugh, make you cry, make you think and then motivate and inspire you to do better. They were the ones with a lot of sobriety—usually decades of sober living. When they were done sharing, they left everyone pondering and contemplating something. Their shares were so deep and thoughtful, but also light and relatable. Whether it was the thought processes of the listeners after, or the quality of the story, no one really liked following a strong share like that.

A homeless-looking guy raised his hand and rambled for a couple of minutes about nothing in particular. He said something about being a millionaire decades before and not needing money, and then went out for a cigarette. The sober alcoholics he left in his wake looked around and rolled their eyes, smiling politely. He would come around here and there, sometimes leave after five minutes, and sometimes fall asleep. Sometimes he would get angry and get up and sit in the corner and murmur to himself. Whatever happened, he would make sure he got a couple of hot dogs, some coffee, and handfuls of cookies. He never donated to the basket but no one ever cared. Sometimes he could be entertaining. Sometimes he could be annoying or downright rude. Sometimes we were just glad we weren't in his shoes at the moment. Whatever happened with him, we were happy he was there. As long as he was breathing there was hope, and the fact that he would show up meant that he was only one day away from getting sober. We prayed for him.

We stood outside and talked for a few minutes and then everyone went their separate ways. The guys from Boston had to get back to the office. Lonnie would give Fred a ride across the river. My friend Jasper would go back to the house he was painting. The homeless guy would surely go to some busy street and ask for money, and I would go play nurse at a nursing home. It was still so new that I just couldn't believe I was a nurse. I was responsible for the lives of so many people. Less than three weeks earlier I had been a waiter at a restaurant downtown, making sure food orders were entered and carried out correctly. My biggest fear was bringing an over-cooked steak back and having to apologize profusely and hope and pray the mistake didn't affect my tip. Now I had to hope and pray that I would know what to do and how to respond if someone had a myocardial infarction on my watch. Life finally got real and one day at a time was the *only* way I could handle it.

I waited for the bus on the corner, not one block from the meeting, and was able to catch the 1:45 bus heading back to my neighborhood. As it rolled into its designated stretch of asphalt next to the curb, I identified Lena as the driver. She was Colombian and had a funny accent that reminded me of Sophia Vergara. I had to put my bike on the front bike cart which was a complicated process. You had to find a lever and press it to release the lock and pull the six-foot-long cart down into its place. Then you had to carefully place both tires in small grooves where you would pull a retractable lock over them to keep the bike in place. The cart only allowed two bikes but I never ran into a problem with bicycle cart occupancy. I was a professional at getting the cart down into position, loading the bike, locking it, and paying my fare. I could do all of this in fifteen seconds. The first time took a little longer and the bus driver had to direct me with hand motions through her enormous windshield. Learning was incredible and many took it for granted. I thought about how long it first took me and how after a couple of times I could do it with my eyes closed. We constantly overlook everyday tasks and can't see the amount of learning that goes into them. I loved riding the bus for many reasons. The schedules were sporadic but thanks to the NJ Transit app I was able to see when the next busses were due in. The app was seldom inaccurate and I was grateful for that—I'd put that on my next gratitude list. I was also grateful for the bus drivers who always helped me when I was new to the bussing culture. They also let me slide sometimes when I was short money or didn't have my app working to pay for the trip. Eventually, I bought a monthly bus pass that would also allow me one-stop train rides, all of this for less than fifty dollars a month. I often contemplated never driving again and relying on public transportation and my bike… but that was eight years away and I was only doing that *one day at a time* thing. On top of all the convenience the bus provided, I always enjoyed the other common folk I would run into. I would sometimes run into people from my Alcohol Support Groups, people from the gym, and other regulars with whom I'd made an acquaintance. Every other ride I was helping old ladies with their bags or explaining to them how much the fare was. Although I suspected the bus drivers appreciated this, my helping others meant I was the real victor. Service to others is how I and many other sober alcoholics survived and thrived. I even got to the point where I could help the driver load riders in wheelchairs through a complicated mechanical lift. We would have to clear out the front of the bus and its passengers and then fold its specialized seats up against the window. The driver would lock some mechanisms and release others, and strap the back wheels of the wheelchair in. I know everyone on the bus was grateful for my help when these handicapped riders came aboard because two sets of hands were better than one and in the tristate, timing and punctuality were everything. On our route, there was also a community center for the blind, so I would always get to see the blind living their life… maybe just a little slower than others. Some of the blind riders had seeing-eye dogs, and I loved dogs so that was also a plus. I couldn't pet the dogs or even talk to them since they were working, but they were fun to look at. Seeing the blind almost daily made me grateful I had all my senses. I also had both hands and feet and all ten fingers and toes. My mini gratitude list for the day—or maybe just the hour—was complete. Thank you, God.

The bus stopped right in front of the dentist's office where I lived above. Sometimes I would forget to pull the bell, but the driver knew where I had to get off and always remembered to stop for me. I locked my bike up out front, knowing I'd be back down in a half-hour, and on the way to work, so the chance of a thief coming up to the busy office with bolt cutters was slim. I chose a Coheed and Cambria playlist on my Spotify app, unplugged the headphones at the bottom of my stairs and by the time I hit the second floor my phone had already connected to the blue tooth speaker and was blaring one of my favorite bands. I hit the shower, and got ready.

I put on my navy blue scrubs from top to bottom. I wore a white bandana. I put my sunglasses back on because of my photosensitivity to light, especially when the light refracted off of car windshields and shiny paint jobs. I wore a light Puma warm-up over my scrub top and no long johns under my scrub pants. It got hot in the nursing home because the elderly were forever cold and always blasting the heat, so I would have to endure slightly chilly bike rides back and forth so I wouldn't overheat during eight hours of labor. I had my backpack with a large water jug and a tall slim canteen for coffee. It also contained my stethoscope and several writing utensils. I also had my wallet and phone in the pack. My headphones ran from my phone in the backpack to my ears, fueling my bike ride.

I went back downstairs, side-stepped a resident at the pay window of the dentist's waiting room, and went out the front door. Leaving for work, I didn't have to worry about locking the front door because the office staff would lock up when they left a couple of hours later. I shot a silent acknowledgment to the office personnel and they shot a nod and a side-smile back.

It was still sunny but it sure was chilly. As I was ready to curse the cold weather, I saw my bike and realized I should be grateful it was still there and nothing else really mattered; my aluminum alloy horse was ready to ride. I would have to reopen my gratitude list and add some more things I was grateful for! On Addison Ave, in order to make the train, I had to bike the 1.5 miles to downtown because the bus schedules just didn't coordinate with the train schedule. If I took an early bus I'd wait thirty minutes on the train platform to be forty-five minutes early to work. If I took the later bus, I wouldn't make it to work on time. I could keep my blood pumping, listen to music, and weave in and out of traffic—safely—after all, I didn't have health insurance yet. I also enjoyed waiting on the train platform. Watching all the different people coming and going. I would turn off the music and call a couple of people from my network of sober folk. One of them was my sponsor who, after a year and a half of sobriety still requested that I call him every single day. This wasn't very common for people who have been sober this long. Many other newly sober persons would call their sponsor once or twice a week. Some newly sober wouldn't call their sponsor at all unless they had a situation that needed perspective or feedback. While waiting on the platform the express train passed by and this was the time for my therapeutic anger outlet. My brother did the same thing. As the train passed at high speeds it got very loud. My brother and I took the opportunity to scream at the top of our lungs and get any frustration or stress out. Normally someone screaming as loud as they would surely attract attention and maybe garner a psychiatric consult. When the express train zipped through, no one could hear you scream which is why it was the perfect time to let any angst and anger out. The next train came minutes later and I got on. I whipped out my phone with my monthly pass. Nine times out of ten the conductor didn't even get to me because my trip is so short. If only I could work out a deal where I didn't pay for the busses, maybe I wouldn't have to pay for any transportation—but that would be dishonest and I was trying to get away from that behavior. I'd been pretty good thus far.

We crossed the bridge over the river and I stood to enjoy the favorite part of my ride. It only lasted six seconds but the views down the calm river were a beautiful sight to behold. Another two minutes and we arrived at Norwich train station. I got out and rode my bike the length of the train and its platform to the overpass over the busy road, crossed it, got off of my bike as it was still rolling, picked it up, and hurried down the stairs. I rode on the sidewalk, which was just redone so it was smoother than the road—and safer. Safety was always at the front of my mind because of that non-existent health insurance. After ninety days of employment I could sign up for health insurance through the union I would then be a part of. My earbuds blasted Matisyahu's Live at Stubb album. Between the cardiac pump I was getting from the bike ride and the instant energy I was getting from my headphones, I was ready to start the shift. I also had twenty ounces of diluted black coffee to take at 1700 to keep my energy level up. Since I'd left early to catch the train, I now had fifteen minutes before clocking in. I sat on a bench next to a poor excuse for a pond, which was designed and intended for the residents. There was also seating on the side of the building with chess board tables, but I never saw anyone outside at either place—maybe because it was winter. *Silly me.* I breathed deeply. I meditated. I prayed. I went over the gratitude list again. As the February chill set in and permeated my Puma warm up jacket, I made my way inside.

When I came to the automatic sliding double doors, I used the Jedi hand sweep to open the automatic door. Perfectly timed, the door opened. I still do this with automatic sliding doors and it never gets old— it always makes me laugh in my head.

I said hello to the front desk secretary and headed to the middle of the building on the second floor. The large nursing station at 2C (2 Central) was always home to two or more nurses and a handful of CNAs sitting during the change of shift. I said hello to all my friends, complimented someone's hair—who was flattered that I noticed— and arrived at the nursing office to confirm my assignment. Luckily, I was back on 2B. The supervisor stated that most likely it would be my permanent assignment. My home. It was a lot easier to have an assigned floor because you got to know all your residents better and they, you. You could also consistently organize and take care of your med-cart, your med-room, your utility room, and your desk.

I walked the hundred yards to my corner where the long hall met the shorter one, to *my* nursing station. As always it was hustling and bustling with residents, staff, linen carts, and random equipment. I decided to call it the hot corner. I'd think of former New York Met and captain David Wright every time I did. I cleaned off a corner next to the fax machine with antiviral, antibacterial, anti-everything wipes. These wipes killed everything—SARS, HIV, Hepatitis, flu—absolutely everything in minutes. I listened and looked around a bit while I was cleaning to get a feel for the unit. It was never good if you heard screams for help when entering the unit but if it was a little too quiet, you had to be skeptical. I heard nothing out of the ordinary and put my backpack down in my newly sanitized area right next to the fax machine. I fetched my green pen, my black pen, my highlighter, and my sharpie. The green pen was for signing the MAR, denoting second shift medications. The black pen was for writing official doctor orders and other notes and reminders to myself. The highlighter was for discontinued orders in the MAR— you could get through the two hundred plus pages faster that way. The sharpie was for writing the date on each newly-opened medication bottle. You could also mark your wound treatment dressings, oxygen cannulas, transdermal patches, piston syringes for G-tube residents, and a number of other things. Date—time—initials. Very important stuff. Preparation and organization were paramount in healthcare and possibly more important in this disorganized and unprepared nursing home. If you had no respect for either you didn't stand a chance of doing any quality work in a timely manner.

I got some scrap paper from the fax machine, making sure there was no resident-sensitive information, for fear of a HIPPA (privacy laws) violation. I folded over a fax receipt and made it my canvas for note-taking during another grueling shift working with these poor souls.

I took report from Tanya and tried to ask important questions and gain information that would help me later. The only relevant thing was a stat blood draw for a PT/INR level on Mr. Cramer. Apparently, they had missed the early a.m. draw and would be back later. I formed a timeline in my head while we opened the narcotic box. I would need the blood drawn by 18:00 to get the results by 20:00 to page the doctor at 20:10 and wait for a call back by 20:30 and then page the doctor again to ultimately get in touch with them by 20:50 at the latest, to administer the Warfarin by 21:00. Tom Brady always got kudos for clock management—the commentators never shut up about his excellence at clock management. I wish Tom could see me planning all this shit out! All narcotics were accounted for. I signed for the cart—now all the narcotics were my responsibility. Tanya took no time to get the heck out of Dodge. I looked up from locking the narc box and then the cart, to see the back of her, halfway down the hundred-yard hallway, walking at a brisk pace. *Nice talking to you too! Yes, I had a good night last night, everything was smooth, thanks for asking!* When it was time to go, you had to hustle out of there before someone caught you to ask a favor, so I didn't blame her.

I checked all the passengers on my manifest to make sure they were all breathing and in no immediate danger. They were all alive and no one had fallen out of their bed, electrocuted themselves, or choked on something. This shift went pretty smoothly. I had to mediate an argument about what TV was being watched in the resident lounge and suddenly understood how my parents felt when me and my siblings would squabble over something as silly as TV time.

The phlebotomist came around 18:00 and drew the blood with no problem. I checked an hour later and the labs were back. I paged the MD and got a call back within the hour. I reported the labs to the MD, wrote the new order in black pen, signed off on it in the MAR in green ink, and put it all to bed. For once, my time and planning actually panned out. "Look at me now, Tawmm!" I shouted in my best Boston accent. My CNA Madeline heard me and poked her head from behind her linen cart, confused.

"'Oo is this Tom? We got new resident?"

"No no, sorry Madeline, never mind. Thank you." I laughed out loud and Madeline probably thought I was crazy. Many of the CNAs enjoyed watching the new nurses stay afloat during the first weeks of their careers. I enjoyed my solo inside joke as well as my Boston accent.

I had about twenty minutes of desk work and rest time before I counted the narcotics and gave report. I also enjoyed a twenty-minute break in-between my 17:00 and 21:00 medication pass. I felt relief and maybe a little bit of triumph. I shaved off more time on both med-passes and was able to laugh a little bit more this shift. Things got a little faster and easier as I went on. Learning was fun for me and extremely beneficial for a new nurse. I was on my way back home in no time. I got home, quietly undressed, and showered. I crept into bed trying not to wake Candace. I said my prayers with an emphasis on gratitude and fell asleep moments after.

Chapter 4

February/March

To rest on your laurels

The next couple of weeks or so went by with no real news to report. I worked out, I went to Alcohol Support Group meetings, and I went to my weekly Board of Nursing meetings to let them know I was still sober and healthy. I went to work five days a week. I went to sleep. Life was good and for the first time in my life, I saw my bank account grow significantly. I made the same money as an LPN as I did as a waiter at a four-star family restaurant, but I had fewer expenses at the moment. A month before, I'd made the last payment on my three-year DWI surcharge penalty of $3,000. I had also paid off a $4,000 hospital bill from the summer before. It had nothing to do with alcoholism, though I was drinking then; I had contracted Rocky Mountain Fever during a birding trip into New York.

I spent no money on drugs or alcohol anymore. I had no car insurance, car payment, or gasoline to pay for. I also didn't have to pay for the bad decisions I always made while drinking; ordering take-out food in a drunken stupor, impulse buying, car repairs, paying bar tabs, paying for drinks for others (we called that bigshot-ism in my Alcohol Support Groups). I was proud of myself for all of my accomplishments and for turning my life around. I was still sober and doing a pretty important job. I was finally, truly contributing to my community and society. My friends from Alcohol Support Groups were also proud of me. I got the claps I yearned for and expected from my sober buddies. Later on in those meetings and without fail, an old-timer would tell a story and lesson about resting on your laurels. "Resting on your laurels" meant that you had achieved certain goals and accomplishments and because of them, you might believe you beat alcohol or didn't need meetings or prayer. You'd become overconfident and stop doing the things that got you sober. Eventually, you would relapse. You had to live your sober life the same way you did when you first got sober. Make meetings, help others, and pray. There were a lot of contradictory statements and opinions in Alcohol Support Groups but you couldn't try to understand them, or take one side—you had to take what you needed and just keep attending. Life was good. I just couldn't take it for granted or think that "I got this" because I would be destined to screw up again if I started thinking like that.

I was able to squeeze in a four-day weekend trip to Arizona with Candace to see my best friend and his fast-growing family. I notified my facility about this trip during my hiring interview, and they allowed me to take it. During the flight there, I saw exactly two people wearing masks because of the silly Coronavirus gaining media attention. These people were worried about nothing, I thought. I had been hearing about the Coronavirus since January. Much like all the other SARS viruses that came and went, I figured the ERs would get a spike in flu-like symptoms residents, but no one would be affected. On Instagram, I saw a post showing that during every election year a new virus made its way around the globe causing panic and anxiety. This reaffirmed my thoughts about how insignificant this CORONA thing would be—but what if this was the one that would be equivalent to the plagues back in the 1800s and a third of our population would be wiped out?! I trusted in God, kept my faith and kept living… one day at a time. No matter the severity or the spread of the Corona flu I would still be working at my facility in New Jersey.

My trip to Arizona was a wonderful one. We got to see Alexander and his wife Brittany. They had four kids—one twelve-year-old and triplets who were less than three years old. They were all so darn well behaved that I recommended they write a book on child-rearing, though I knew nothing about the subject. I asked them what the secret was and they told me *consistency*. I told them that was the same approach I used with my sobriety! We laughed and then I told them my plans to go to a meeting in the morning at seven a.m. I asked if I could borrow a bicycle so as not to trouble anyone with a ride.

The following day I rode through the desert to get my spiritual fix. The sun was coming over the mountains as I made my way towards the church. There were cacti and other strange plants in the forefront of the mountains. It was almost as if I was on another planet. I thought of scenes from the original Star Trek and wondered if they were filmed out here. The sun was glorious that day. Some of my fellow sober people called such a scene a "God Moment." I met a dozen strangers inside the church at 7:30 a.m., sipping coffee and shooting the shit. I had just met all of them, but it was like we were old friends reuniting after ten years. We all could relate to each other and that's why it worked so well. I told them I'd see them at the next meeting and we went about our day. They were all going to work whereas I was headed back to vacationing with my friends. When I got back to the house, Arthur pulled me aside and asked, "Hey are you okay, man? Do you want me to not drink in front of you?!" He questioned me with great concern.

"Haha!" I laughed out loud in front of him, which confused him. "No my friend, thank you for thinking of me though. I just like going to meetings, I feel great after them. I truly haven't had a desire to drink since getting sober almost two years ago. Drink up, my brother!" I said confidently while still skeptical of my life's new trajectory. *Is this my real life? Why didn't I do this sooner? Why didn't anyone tell me sober life could be so full and fun!?* Alexander drank whiskey that night, the girls had wine, and I had seltzer. It didn't bother me. We had another night in Arizona and I got to one more meeting with my new family I'd never met but knew so well. It was a great trip and I was ready to come back to New Jersey to resume my brand new career.

We saw another fool in a mask in the airport on the way back. I quickly judged the person, but then thought maybe the person had a cold and didn't want to infect anyone else, which was actually quite thoughtful. In many parts of Asia, this was a common practice when one was feeling under the weather. They would wear masks anywhere and everywhere when they weren't feeling well.

Candace and I got back to the tristate safely and ready to get back to work. I had worked on my tan and everyone noticed and commented on it. During the winters here everyone was really pale, so when you went somewhere and brought a tan back, you stuck out like a sore thumb.

Every day on the cart went a little faster and smoother. If you do something repeatedly long enough you will become a professional at it. The truth was that a monkey could hand out all these pills to the right residents if the monkey had enough practice. My *brain-med-cart* connections were strengthening and before flipping the pages of the MAR I knew who would be the next resident and what I had to do for them. I started to anticipate where in the cart their medication was located and where their eye drops and nasal sprays might be. I remembered from the day before, which of the medications were running low and had to be re-ordered. I learned the schedules of the CNAs, which rooms they would be in at what times, and how to avoid getting in their way. I could predict the precise time when the sundowning would start to affect the brains of my elderly inmates; I would get in there when they would start to cry and worry and I'd talk quickly to distract them. I would ask them questions furiously and then answer my own questions just as quickly in a similar way Vince Vaughn spoke in Wedding Crashers. They went from worried to entertained to intrigued. I would end with a promise to return soon after. I hoped all the information, interaction, and stimuli I had just provided them, would keep their mind focused on solving a mystery as to who I was and what I was doing, until I could return. If they focused on those things they would be less likely to concentrate on getting out of their bed and taking the walk of faith… at least for a couple more minutes. I would then come back and wave and might get a smile in return. Sometimes they would stare at me blankly and I thought nothing would work on certain residents.

During this time I also learned which CNAs could be trusted and counted on. I learned which ones might neglect a resident and leave someone sitting in their own waste. I had to check certain residents at the end of the shift and if I found them sitting in their own excrement I would quickly tell the CNA to change them before the end of their shift. They eventually got used to this. Some responded positively and made sure all the work was done, while others enjoyed waiting for the cat and mouse game we would play. They would take the chance of me finding incomplete work and then having to find the CNA who would have to complete the work. When I spoke to experienced nurses about the CNAs and their work habits, they said things like: CNA school teaches them to hide, or that CNA was short for Certainly Never Around. They saw how hard I worked and most of them took a liking to me. I would also help them with whatever they needed whenever they asked. I kept learning more and more about the residents and CNAs and they kept learning about me.

As some things clicked and I revised and refined everything about my practice, the shifts were filled with curveballs and unpleasant surprises. For someone whose life was only holding on by habit and routine, this was extremely difficult. I could do all my pre-work rituals in the same order every day, but as soon as I entered those facility doors, all of that could be thrown to the wind. Anything could and would happen and it certainly flustered me. The only thing that I could keep organized and routine was the order in which I said my prayers. That was my lifeline and no one could take it from me.

The Corona thing had a new name. COVID-19 was gaining momentum and popularity. During the beginning of March, it was all I heard about. I thought eventually the press and interest would die down and we'd get back to spring cleaning and spring training. *Boy, was I wrong...*

...

The New York state of emergency was called on March seventh; the New Jersey counterpart was on March ninth, but I still wasn't too worried. Even with the Stay and Shelter orders, I continued on with life because I was considered essential personnel and believed that it was all much ado about nothing. Even after the president called it a national emergency on March thirteenth I was more entertained than worried. The general population would have to humor our local and federal government's wishes until we could come out of our houses. Many of the stores in the tristate were closed down except for convenience stores, liquor stores, and grocery stores. People still had to eat and drink. People also still needed to shit. Toilet paper almost became a valuable form of currency since there was none to be found in the early days of the COVID. All the world was panicking for toilet paper, just like inmates would in prison or jail. Despite the Stay and Shelter, Candace and I took walks outside as her cabin fever set in. She would drive me to and from work since the trains weren't running and I paid her money to do so. It was a form of income for her since she wasn't allowed to work and it got her outside the house a couple of times a day. I called her my Corona Uber. I left my ID badge in her car so that if the police pulled her over, she could show that she was transporting essential personnel—suddenly my self-importance grew. My life and lifestyle up until this time had been anything but essential.

I remember the day and time after Rudy Gober of the Utah Jazz tested positive for the virus, and when the commissioner of the NBA, Adam Silver officially suspended the 2019-2020 season indefinitely. All those broadcasters speculating that if the season ended today, the playoff bracket would be such and such… was actually going to happen! I remember hearing the news from Agatha Monroe's TV set. I was in the hall preparing her medications and I stepped in to have a listen and confirm what I'd heard. I started to panic and thought to myself, *What if this was really it?! The end of the world! What would I do? Might as well drink and party till my time comes!* The NBA was going to cancel the rest of the season and forfeit millions, if not billions, of dollars! Could it be this serious?! I immediately reflected how I hadn't been as worried when I'd heard of tristate emergencies, but when the almighty NBA pulled the plug on their season, I really started to take it seriously. I let the thoughts run around in my head for a couple of seconds before I shut down my negative, unproductive thinking and focused on the task at hand. God was too good to let the world come to an end, but I still pondered the outcome. To my knowledge, no one in the facility had the virus. No one I knew outside the facility had the virus. I decided to focus on what I had in front of me; another twelve residents who needed their 21:00 medications. The antidote to fear is faith. My faith in God was strong and I decided to keep helping those in need. After all, *Faith without Works is dead.*

I don't really remember getting home that night; my mind wandered here and there and I contemplated where and when and who and why. I do remember Candace waiting outside for thirty minutes because I got out of work late. My guilt for Candace and for making her wait overtook the worry and concern about the global panic. I tried to stay grounded as best I could, but it looked like the world might be getting very sick, and luckily for me, I got into nursing just in time for a worldwide pandemic.

···

I don't remember exactly when, but we were all issued surgical masks and our facility was locked down. We allowed no visitors. No family was allowed entry. Not even our food vendors or delivery persons were allowed in. Our staff would have to unload the trucks coming in and were to have no contact with the drivers. With such a tight lockdown, I figured our facility was the safest place in the state—no COVID could get through our doors. We had staff stationed at the door with a thermometer gun checking temperatures. They were also armed with a brief set of questions for every employee: in the last twenty-four hours have you had any cough? Have you had any fever? Have you had any shortness of breath? After answering the questions satisfactorily we would grab our surgical masks and get to work. Between the thermometer readings and these questions, none of the infected could possibly enter our facility… I was sure of it! Right!?

Wrong!

...

The previous two weeks hadn't been so bad. Everyone was a little giddy and anxious. We all felt somewhat confident in our viral security force at the front door. I walked in, signed my name, date, and time, and immediately sanitized my hands. The greeters didn't even ask the questions anymore; it was understood that we would tell them if we had any fever, cough, or difficulty breathing. We would also let them know if we had traveled out of state in the last fourteen hours since our last shift the night before. It was almost a joke and no one really took it too seriously. Since no one was allowed in, no COVID could possibly gain entry, either! We worked the same way as if nothing had happened. The only difference was that we were all in surgical masks. We figured the two-week lockdown to flatten the curve would be effective and have everyone back on their feet and living regular lives any day now. That day would be the day we discovered our first COVID case—Evelyn Wolney, an eighty-six-year-old, fully dependent, bed-ridden female. She had the trifecta of diagnoses that we soon learned was the worst for COVID-positive residents—COPD, diabetes, and CHF. She was on my side of the hundred-yard corridor leading to my hall. We didn't have the rapid swab tests yet, but a PCR (a two-day lab test) was available in small amounts and Evelyn was swabbed that morning. Our in-house NP (Nurse Practitioner) diagnosed it as COVID, without knowing for certain. I stood at the desk hearing the report and counting the narcotics as my mind drifted away. Tanya's cheeks and eyes were moving as if she was talking but I wasn't sure because of the mask covering her mouth. I kept thinking of poor Evelyn. I'd only had her as a resident once and she was absolutely delightful. She was very thin and very frail. You had to be careful moving her in bed because you could probably break her bones just by using a little too much force. I remember that she kept reassuring me that I was doing a good job. Somehow she knew that I was a new nurse, and remarked about it frequently, but always in a positive way. I remembered her smiling. She refused to wear her dentures and her mouth looked similar to the way a newborn's would. I remember injecting her with insulin and she made some joke about taking a shot of alcohol or something. I made a mental note to say a prayer for her, once I was done pretending to listen to Tanya. I had to pay more attention while counting the narcs. Tanya filled me in on the Evelyn situation—she was a fan favorite after all.

Evelyn was immediately moved to the newly designated quarantine unit on the first floor. The next question was, who gave COVID to her and how did they get in? She had family who visited sometimes, but no one had been allowed in since March ninth. It was like a *whodunnit* movie; we all started to look at each other and question who might be carrying the viral weapon. If one of us had it, how could we have gotten by our security team of thermometer and questions? Maybe we were asymptomatic. We could be breathing on everyone right now. Right this instant, the virus could be spreading exponentially until the whole building and its inhabitants were doomed. All we could do was to keep our surgical masks on, wash our hands, and hope for the best. Evelyn had been moved downstairs right after lunch. She'd been in a double room but her roommate had passed away three months earlier, and luckily, she hadn't found a new roommate yet. The door was closed and had a 'DO NOT OPEN' sign on it in bright red lettering. At the bottom of the sign it read, 'Management.' I thought about calling my imaginary bookie and taking the *over* on how many times that door would be opened by 23:00. I was confident in my fictitious bet as well as human nature. Most of the folks I worked with ignored rules, regulations, and certainly *bright red signs and exclamation points*. Maybe some of them were illiterate. Some were curious. Some just had to break the rules. I couldn't blame them because I was the same way. Tell me not to push the button and that button was surely going to get pushed.

Now that the virus was in the building, if there was any truth to what the media was saying, it would spread like wildfire, leaving bodies in its trail.

Once Tanya had left, I prayed to God, and really let the worry set in. I pondered how I would go in and out of the rooms touching as few things as I could. I remember that night getting questioned by staff from all over, about what had happened to Evelyn. The gossip certainly spread faster than any virus out there. Some of the rumors were that her roommate had already died this morning from COVID! They were also saying that Evelyn was dead too. It was a warped and morbid game of telephone. It distracted people and kept them from doing their jobs correctly, if at all.

At 20:00 hours I got up from my desk and was about to start my med-pass when I saw an employee open Evelyn's door despite the big red lettering and the stop sign under it. "YO!" I shouted at the top of my lungs. The employee closed the door, backed up, and turned down the hundred-yard hallway towards the middle of the building. He muttered *sorry* while doing so. I was livid—and for the first time ever I comprehended the word livid, and all of its meaning. "THAT'S COVID, MAN!" I yelled in a nicer tone but equally loud voice. I could imagine him opening the door and sucking in little droplet particles of COVID, and breathing out the little particles into every room he passed. All the residents were now on lockdown since the new developments. Most had their doors shut and were literally fearing for their lives. The nurse and the CNA would be the only contact they would have for the next two months.

…

I focused on the task at hand and finished my shift. Since March ninth, with the Stay and Shelter order, no one was on the roads. Everything was eerily empty; the roads, the train, and all the shops and stores were closed, save for a few convenience stores that allowed no one in unless they had a mask. The few who did visit the stores, complied with the mask order. Plastic sheets separated the customer from the cashier. You had to hand everything under the makeshift plastic shower lining they'd hung up—it was better than nothing, I guess.

The trains started to run again for essential personnel so I took them. It kept me and Candace from being in close quarters in the car, which she worried about, now that we had a positive case. I was the only one riding the trains for another month. The conductors were there but not checking tickets for fear of exposure. I stood in the vestibule in between cars because there was airflow and I didn't want to infect any invisible travelers. I also didn't want to leave any COVID on any inanimate objects. My monthly pass was going to waste since they never checked for tickets. The buses were running but I didn't take them because of our mismatching schedules. I had no meetings or gym to get to during this time so I didn't need the bus anyway. I missed Cesar and Lena and hoped they were doing well. The front half of the buses were sectioned off for the bus drivers' safety and they kept the windows open to keep any unwanted organisms from hanging around. It was still chilly out so they had the heat blasting to counter the cold air coming in, but there were hardly any passengers anyway.

When I got home, I was especially careful with my clothes. I took everything off, including my sneakers, and left it all at the bottom of the stairs. I walked up the stairs naked and brought back down a black trash bag to put everything in, except for my shoes. I would leave the trash bag there in hope of keeping my apartment free of the COVID. I would pile the bag up until it was full and bring it to the laundromat down the street. Depending on my schedule, sometimes I would pay for the laundry to be done. They did a good job but it was rather expensive. I would usually treat the laundryman, Paco, to a Dunkin Donuts coffee because he was very kind and quite exceptional at his job. He was so grateful for the coffee. It was totally worth it to be able to make someone's day… for a dollar-fifty. Sometimes I would do the laundry myself, handling it with the utmost care in case there were any COVID particles longing for a living host. It was so early on and no one knew if the virus was actually able to live on inanimate objects and if so, for how long. One day I brought my laundry to my hardworking friend Paco. He greeted me and tried to take my laundry. Paco could tell when someone was new at doing laundry at a laundromat, and he would bounce around and help them. Some might consider his occupation as less important, but he was great at it and proud of what he did. When he approached me to help, he saw the scrubs and halted, and asked in Spanglish, "Tu eres enfermero, my friend?" *(Are you a nurse?)*

"Si Papa…trabajando con el COVID mucho ahora," *(Yes, I work a lot with COVID now)* I retorted quietly so no one else would worry. I liked to keep my lingual skills up to par so he always humored me.

"Oh man, that's gotta be rough, Papa, Dios te bendiga." He said through a sad and sympathetic face. I gathered that he said something about God blessing me so I said,

"Gracias hermano, no olvida a lavar tus manos, Papa," I said, half jokingly. I told him not to forget about washing his hands in my broken but comprehendible Spanish.

"?!Su ropa tiene el Covid?!" *(Your clothes have Covid?)* He asked a little too loudly for my liking. People around us started looking. I literally saw people's faces change when they realized that my bag was full of medical scrubs. No one moved away or tightened their masks but they did surely take notice. I responded quickly and went to work. "No se Papa! Vamos a lavar!" *(I don't know. let's wash!)* I furiously loaded the washer with my weaponized scrubs. I laughed in my head but projected concern for the others in the laundromat who would probably appreciate my speed and caution.

I showered, prayed, and went to bed. I scrubbed extra hard in the shower that night. I paid special attention to my ears and face, thinking there might be remnants of the virus somewhere on my exposed ears. I always tried to exfoliate with some type of loofa or washcloth so that night I scrubbed so hard I thought my skin would fall off. After rinsing I lathered and scrubbed a second time. I wasn't especially scared of COVID but I had to do my part as a nurse to stop the spread. I prayed for all the souls in my facility and the whole world. I prayed for the goodness of human nature to prevail. I prayed for there to be enough toilet paper for everyone. Falling asleep was easy because I was exhausted.

...

The next day we had three more cases. The NP diagnosed all three cases. All had fevers, and they complained of difficulty breathing. Their oxygen saturation readings were still within normal limits (the virus wasn't in full swing yet for these residents). A doctor in the building examined the residents and concurred with the NP's diagnosis—*as if the NP's diagnosis wasn't enough.* Even if it wasn't COVID, we could take no chances—we had to separate and quarantine. The PCRs were pending for these three, as well as Evelyn. We continued to wonder; who brought it in? We had been locked down for over two weeks now. It must have been staff, but who? We began to wonder how many other cases would appear? How fast? Was it spreading right now? Was the whole building doomed? The three other cases were in close proximity to resident zero, Evelyn. One was next door to her room, one diagonally across the hall, and the other case was three doors down. All the rooms were within twenty yards of each other. We hoped the 'outbreak' would be contained in this area. The red signs went up as the doors were closed. No one knew how to proceed. Since two cases or more were considered an outbreak we would have to wear full PPE every shift for the next three months. The PPE was on deck but there weren't enough so the Director of Nursing had to order it by the truckload. The response was pretty quick. Isolation carts were placed outside the rooms of the affected in the quarantine unit. The conference room was turned into the PPE locker room. Right before the beginning of the pandemic, our infection control nurse went out on maternity leave. Her one and only job was to educate and manage infectious disease protocols and practices. She was nowhere to be found during the whole first six months of the pandemic. This was the epitome of irony. As with everything else in my life, I waited for things to play out and I did my job the best I could. Some people caved in these situations. Some people wanted to sit and gossip and forget about their job. Some people kept working and helping those in need. I chose to work. Speculation was worthless to me. I did start to worry, but as soon as I did, I prayed and I kept my faith. If God wanted to take souls, he would. If he wanted to take mine, he would.

Chapter 5

March 26th

It could always be worse - unknown

The next day I tested the check-in and PPE process. I pretended I was a secret shopper or some type of corporate spy to evaluate efficiency and safety in the factory. We sanitized on the way in and signed our names, date, and time. They aimed at our forehead with the thermo-gun. The questions were not asked, some people's temperatures read too low or didn't read at all, but because of the line out the door, they were allowed to be skipped and a false temperature was recorded. I couldn't really blame them and it didn't really bother me, although it should have. My reasoning was that most people were taking their temperature at home anyway and at the first sign of any type of symptom, my coworkers would call out—very few had a decent work ethic and they were always looking for time off. On top of that, we were issued n95 masks to wear under the surgical masks. The n95s were to keep the COVID out of our respiratory tract as well as keep the virus from escaping if it was already within us. The surgical masks were to be worn to keep the n95s clean. We would have to reuse them for as long as possible because of the worldwide shortage. After we donned our double masks, we sanitized our hands and went to the PPE locker room in the first-floor conference room. We stood in line behind the same person as we did in the lobby's viral security station. We got a surgical cap for our head. We got a blue plastic gown. We also got a face shield or goggles. We were also issued booties for our shoes. By this time we had two more cases from the same corridor where the first four were found. Evelyn's

PCR COVID swab came back as positive. The other three were pending, and the next two that had been diagnosed with fever and cough were sent down to the 1A quarantine as well. I learned all this while in the nursing office waiting for my assignment. Surely I would be back on 2B with my regular residents. I waited while the nurses and CNAs before me got their assignments and left. I stepped up and Carrie told me I was to report to 1A quarantine. I was shocked but I didn't question it; I even said thank you and left. I figured they were dealing with enough people giving them grief about COVID assignments, if they didn't refuse the assignment altogether. When you get into health care, you accept the possibility of an epidemic or pandemic happening and the possibility that you could be up close and personal with a dangerous infectious disease.

I walked down the hall to the opposite side of the building towards the quarantine area. I said hello to some residents and some employees. By now, some knew that I was headed to the quarantine unit; one person even wished me luck. I started to fear for my life and almost let panic get the better of me. I took the stairwell down one floor and I wondered why I was chosen. I was a brand new nurse with no experience whatsoever... I knew residents and employees could tell I was intelligent and hardworking. They knew from what they saw so far that I did a pretty good job. Was I more qualified to do this job?! No way! I had been a nurse for barely a month! I was an LPN on top of all that. I had no experience with infectious diseases or much else for that matter. Everyone knew I was a new nurse! I came to the conclusion that it was because of my demographics. I had no wife at home, no children, and was probably one of the younger nurses in the building. I concluded that that's why management chose me. I was the first penguin to test the waters for sharks. None of this really bothered me. If I had walked in here drunk or hung over I might have protested loudly and obnoxiously, but that wasn't me anymore. God had His reasons and mysterious ways and here I was in our COVID unit, ready to do the best job I could.

I entered the unit and decided not to round on the six residents—all of them were breathing, according to Claudia, the RN stationed on the unit. She was a Filipino nurse with tons of experience and little patience. I'd had run-ins with her while she'd been orienting me. During my training with Claudia, she'd offered little help or insight. She let me sink or swim and I took it personally. If I didn't know what an abbreviation meant she would take offense and yell the extended version at me quite condescendingly. *How was I supposed to remember that!? I went to nursing school six years ago, you bitch!* While hours behind on a med-pass she would come to my cart, see where I was and ask why I was so behind, huff and puff and stomp away. After interactions like this, I felt stupid, helpless, and wanting to escape. All the anger built inside and I could do nothing to remedy it. I tried to soldier on and went about the shift and kept communication with her to a minimum. This was another first encounter that all my professors warned me about and I'd refused to believe— "Nurses eat their young." I would find out it was a pandemic all its own. Nursing school is literally all book smarts, then you hit the 'streets' and realize your book smarts can only do so much for you. The 'street smarts' of health care are the more important of the two and having a good nurse orienting you made all the difference in gaining that intangible intelligence.

Report was quick and easy and there was only one narcotic on the floor that needed counting. The one thing I had going for me was a low census (resident count). There were no tracheostomies (artificial air hole through the trachea) to take care of and no G-tubes (gastrostomy tubes) I would have to administer medications through. Three of my residents were full codes and three of them were DNR. A full code means we would have to do everything and anything to revive a dying person and call an ambulance. A DNR was short for Do Not Resuscitate. If the resident was on the way to the other side, we would let them go while doing our best to ensure comfort. Three and three. Split right down the middle. I wondered what the Vegas odds would be on each resident surviving. What would be the *over/under* on deaths? What would be the *over/under* on how long I could survive before I cracked? How about the length of time it would take for each one to pass? The way the media made out this virus, surely two out of three would perish. My orders were to take vital signs twice a shift and administer their medications just like any other day. I would have to take into account infection control. I would go to the one positive case last, in case the others were false positives. This would decrease the chance of infecting them if they didn't really have the COVID.

Claudia left without saying goodbye, and I was no better because I didn't either. I guess I was still salty over the way she had treated me a month ago. I wondered why she would be orienting new nurses when she didn't have the patience for them. She was in no way a teacher or leader. You could be a great nurse but a terrible teacher and that was the case with her. I wondered why she got put down here and if she was angry that she was. I wondered if Claudia and I would bond through this stressful and dangerous assignment. I was alone on the floor until my CNA Mira showed up. Mira blasted through the double doors with her linen cart a full two feet taller than she was. She was yelling non-stop. Some in English, but mostly in French. The only words in English I could make out was "bull shee." We had worked together a couple times so I tried to talk to her and calm her down. I tried to share my positive outlook and force it upon her but there was no chance of any positivity rubbing off. She was all worked up that she drew the shortest straw. I remember her saying how she had a husband and three daughters.

"Dis no good, why they put me down here?!" she yelled at me, trying to contain herself, but I could see her eyes welling up behind the face shield she wore.

"I'm sorry Mira, we just have to be very smart and very careful and we should be fine," I said in a loud but calm voice. I knew she spoke English very well, but because of her angry and frantic state she would not be the best listener. I repeated this again, slowing down when I came to the words *smart* and *careful* and emphasizing them. I told her to sit down and breathe, but by this time her tears were rolling quickly down her face. She wasn't ready to talk so I took the silence as my cue, and improvised as best I could. "We're going to be in and out very quick; no one will know we were there. You know—like navy SEALs?" I asked her, expecting her to know nothing of our covert ops teams.

"Yes, zee military" she laughed and took off her face shield to wipe her tears away.

I told her to breathe again. *COVID unit and I gotta babysit and give pep talks now.* "Yes, exactly! Just breathe and relax, okay? I just checked on all the residents, they're all fine. I'll help you change them so we can be quicker and we'll get through this. I'll be right back. Just breathe, Mira! Navy SEALs!" I tried to assure her, but I really didn't know if we would be okay. It was in God's hands as always. She didn't see my military salute as

I walked quickly down the hall, as if to check on something, but secretly, just giving her some time to gather herself.

I walked to the empty end of the hall and into vacant room. I said the Serenity Prayer followed by the Our Father. My eyes filled with tears. I said the other Alcohol Support Group prayers. I pulled it together and said out loud, "It's not that bad." This was my go-to phrase during stress and adversity. That, or "It could always be worse." I took a couple deep breaths and figured I would *actually* check on all six souls on the manifest as I made my way back to headquarters.

Mira was talking on the phone, to family, I presumed, because it was all French. I'd forgotten to pray for her. I said a quick one in my head as I passed the nursing station where she sat. I gave her a thumbs up and waited for her to reply. She looked up and gave me a one-handed wave and continued her conversation. I got to my med-cart and kept wondering why Mira and I got selected for this dance of death. I couldn't find any reasoning for this. They didn't go by seniority or experience. They didn't go by whether or not we had family. Did they go by intelligence? Physical attributes? Religion practiced? Favorite food? Blood type? Horoscope sign!? I passed on asking her birthday while trying to make light of the situation in my head. Did they literally draw straws? Pick out of a hat? They couldn't have picked employees who were least likely to make a stink, because they wouldn't have chosen Mira. She had a temper and was very outspoken and everyone in the building knew that. Maybe it was punishment for her loud mouth. Nothing ever made sense in this building so far. You add a pandemic to the mix and this place was sure to implode. In this building, reason and rationale were never anywhere to be found. The only thing that made sense was that nothing ever made sense.

By this time our maintenance department had set up negative pressure isolation fans in all the rooms—twenty-eight of them to be exact. They must have contracted someone or gotten help because the maintenance department was only one person. Isaac, an athletic six-foot-two kid, worked pretty fast, but not fast enough to install all twenty-eight fans. The fans worked great, though. They would draw the air from the rooms to the outside of the building, preventing particles from leaking into the hallways and infecting the rest of the building. The doors were to be kept shut. The isolation carts were outside each room. We would put an additional gown on before entering to keep our permanent gown clean, then take off the gown and gloves at the door, before exiting into the hallway.

It was time to check the MAR and see what I was in for. The MAR was extremely thin and the large med-cart was completely empty. I was accustomed to a fat MAR filled with hundreds of pages and a med-cart bursting with bingo cards. It was an utter relief to have so few contents in both places but somehow I also found it depressing.

I was able to do my 1700 med-pass pretty quickly. I also did full vital signs on everyone. I paid special attention to each resident's temperature and oxygen saturation. These two things were most important in the resident's status. If a fever got too high, it was dangerous. If the oxygen saturation got too low, it was dangerous. For fever, all we could do was give Tylenol every six hours. For hypoxia, (low oxygen in the blood) we would administer oxygen through a nasal cannula. If the nasal cannula couldn't help the resident maintain a 95% oxygen rate, we would try a non-rebreather mask at 15 liters per minute. If that didn't work, we would send the resident to the hospital. If the resident was a DNR, we would do our best to keep them breathing. If nothing worked, we would let the resident go to the other side. We were instructed not to send residents to the ER, but to do the best we could with what we had. The hospital beds were scarce and were better off used for younger residents with their whole lives ahead of them, rather than the already sick and diseased elderly. The rationale reminded me of the Normandy scene in Saving Private Ryan. The medic was scurrying frantically across the beach triaging who could be saved and who couldn't. The ones that couldn't be saved would get morphine to help them cross to the other side easier and keep them free from pain. The ones that had a shot at living would get medical attention while under fire.

That night there was only one fever. It was 101.3 and was the first fever I or the resident had encountered in this new age of quarantine, isolation and pandemic. I gave Tylenol and water and instructed the resident to make no fuss and take them both because he had the virus and we didn't know how his body would react. All six of my resident's oxygen saturations were 95% or better. They were all in good spirits, considering the circumstances.

I helped the CNA Mira with one brief change because the resident was confused, combative, and obese. This was his normal behavior so we didn't attribute it to the COVID. I told her I would help her with all of them so we could do it faster but she didn't ask for any other help. I got a laugh when I mentioned the Navy Seals again, and speed. Maybe laughter *was* the best medicine. I always offered to help the CNAs to show them I was willing to work, but they never asked for help and did the job anyway.

I started my 2100 med-pass around 2000 and it went smoothly. With nursing when there is a problem, you have to implement an intervention. The problem was fever. The intervention was Tylenol. After implementing the intervention you then had to evaluate whether or not the intervention was effective. I took the resident's temperature and it came down to 99.1. Still a little high, but it was two degrees less than when I'd checked it five hours ago. In another hour I could give another dose of Tylenol to try to keep the fever at bay. I completed the rest of the vital signs and everyone was doing just fine. I finished the medications.

I brought water to those who needed it. After six hours of donning and doffing PPE every time I entered a room, I got tired of it real quick. When dropping off the water I hustled in and out, holding my breath and opening and closing the door quickly. I listened to every resident's lung sounds and they all sounded clear. I charted in each resident's chart and cleaned up the desk a little. I set my phone alarm for 2200, at which time I would check the resident's temperature again and administer Tylenol. This time, it read 99.9 degrees. It had gone up 0.8 degrees in an hour. I wasn't too worried about the fever. I had confidence in acetaminophen's antipyretic effects. I gave the Tylenol and told the resident to keep drinking water: "You're sick and you need the Tylenol and the water. You have a virus!" I said "a virus" because I didn't want to give any more power to the COVID by calling it "*the* virus." The resident, Jerard Hennessey, seemed to understand. He also understood the magnitude of the virus. He was one of the newsies who watched CNN all day, every day. He was not worried. At one point he told me that he'd lived a long and full life and if it was his time, he would have no fear. I admired his faith. I took it with me as I left his room, and said, "See you tomorrow my friend! Keep drinking that water!"

"God willing!" He chuckled as I closed the door.

Damn! The world is freaking out and he's sitting here with the virus in full swing and he's cool as a fucking cucumber. God bless him.

I sat down and charted the second dose of Tylenol I'd just given. I wrote it in the twenty-four-hour report. It was the only thing I had to report to the oncoming nurse, who turns out, was forty minutes late. I didn't ask or care why she was late, but I figured she was protesting her death sentence of an assignment. Everyone did. Everyone except me. I followed orders whether I liked it or not. I knew the risks when I got into nursing. Infectious diseases were a part of it and every professor let us know on the first day of nursing school. I thought of the nerve of some nurses who had refused the assignment or had refused to come to work altogether. I wanted to curse them all but figured doing so would be "NUT". Negative, Unproductive Thinking. It would be a toxic waste of time. I also considered how I was certainly in no position to judge.

I gave my short report and told the oncoming nurse to keep an eye on Jerard and his fever, happy to report that he was in good spirits. A positive mentality in a time like this went a very long way. I was also happy to report there was no oxygen desaturation in the whole unit. This was great news to hear for the oncoming nurse. A fever could be treated with Tylenol, but once you get into breathing difficulty, that's when it got scary and you really had to work to keep the resident above ground. You learn what type of nurse you are when a resident says they can't breathe. What do you do first? What equipment do you grab? What vital signs are the priority? Who do you call? When do you call them? I equated an eight-hour nursing shift to a game of Russian roulette or maybe Jenga. Now with a deadly respiratory virus, the game became much more serious. Even after the best nurse implemented every preventative measure it would come down to luck and chance and you just wanted to get out of there after your eight hours, without incident. The oncoming nurse would then wait out their eight hours, and it would go on and on.

I wished my night nurse good luck and walked out with Mira. We did a sort of debriefing on our walkout. She kept complaining about why her, and never again, and all sorts of other negative, self-pity talk. She never once asked about me. I didn't mind. God gave me another chance in life and maybe this was why. I got this job a month before the Pandemic. I had nothing to do with healthcare a year ago. I told her to have faith in God and that maybe He would keep her safe. I couldn't say for certain whether God intended to keep Mira around or not. I told her she served her country well and saluted her again. We parted ways and she skeptically saluted me back. "Tank you, David, Gah bless you 'unny" she said walking to the parking lot. *I should get paid for these kinds of talks. Maybe I'll get into motivational speaking when I'm done with this…*

I unlocked my bike and rode the empty roads to the train station. I climbed the stairs and waited on the empty platform. The train came minutes later. It was empty. I took my six-minute ride back to the city I lived in and rode towards home. Addison Avenue was completely empty. I would see a cop driving through here and there. One actually shined his light on me the first week of the shutdown. He saw I was in navy blue scrubs and turned it off. I thought it was funny that the police and I were now friends. I made it home, undressed, and threw my dirty scrubs in the dirty trash bag. I tied it in a loose knot and left it at the bottom of the stairs. I showered, prayed, and went to bed. Candace was fast asleep so she didn't know I'd been the COVID nurse that night…

Chapter 6

March 27th

One day at a time

I woke up, greeted Candace with a kiss on the cheek, and played my music loudly. I started to make breakfast for the two of us and wondered why she hadn't made some for us already. The music was blaring and Candace seemed uncomfortable with it so I changed it to Dave Matthews Band, knowing she would enjoy that better. The dentists hadn't been in the office for over two weeks now. I had a very large speaker that I could let fire away when the dentists weren't around. We played Dave Matthews Band at about 75% of the speaker's full potential. I cooked our breakfast and danced around a bit in the kitchen where Candace couldn't see me. Once I had the music going and some coffee in me, my grateful mood got even better, even if the whole world was crashing and burning. After a while, I turned the music down a little bit and put on Dispatch. Dispatch was my favorite band and it would always get me through tough times. I sat next to Candace and we ate scrambled eggs with peppers and onions. I made some toast and put peanut butter on it. It was a pretty healthy breakfast. I opened a fresh bottle of Stop & Shop Raspberry Seltzer. They had *the best* selection of seltzer and they were only forty-nine cents for a thirty-two-ounce bottle. I knew all about seltzer now. Every sober alcoholic does. Coffee and Seltzer. We turned the TV on and browsed Netflix and saw something about a Tiger King. I'd heard about it at work. I also saw some posts on Instagram about it. People seemed to love it and were vastly entertained by the mini-series. I mentioned to Candace how I had been stationed on the COVID unit and she was not too pleased. It was as if a record skipped when someone who didn't belong walked into the room. She put down her magazine and looked at me with wide eyes. I could tell her brain was processing her own risk and exposure. I talked to her and tried to comfort her the best I could. I told her I was extremely careful and I had full PPE on the whole time while in the quarantine unit. I told her how vigorously I had been scrubbing in the shower and how thorough I was when brushing my teeth. This seemed to ease her mind a bit but she still took to cleaning every surface multiple times a day.

We turned off the music and started to watch the Tiger King. We got one episode in and we were hooked. At this point, I would have been going to the gym and then to a meeting, but the whole world was closed. I had been going to the gym and meetings six out of seven days, every week for over a year and a half. The thought of being deprived of my physical, mental, and spiritual relief depressed me. I looked out the window onto Addison Avenue. There was no one. The 7-11 across the street had sporadic customers here and there. Some were on foot. Some were on bikes. Very few cars were on the road yet. Folks were saying that the reduced emissions and reduced waste were doing wonders for the environment. I couldn't tell, but I hoped it was true. I do recall my brother-in-law telling me he'd taken his dog to the Jersey shore and had seen a seal hanging out on the beach. I'd had never seen a seal on any Jersey shore. I guess the aquatic ecosystem and its inhabitants appreciated the absence of humans on their beaches. Everything was beginning to depress me but I kept in mind, that maybe mother nature needed some time to heal her wounds and breathe some clean air.

I got right back to the couch where Candace was reading her magazine in between episodes and we watched another episode of the Tiger man. By this time I was a week or two late to the tiger party. After all, I had to keep working while the rest of the world enjoyed weeks off on the couch. After the next episode, I did 150 push-ups and 150 sit-ups and then got right back to the couch. Body weight exercises weren't my thing but it was better than nothing. We couldn't finish the third episode, because I was scheduled to work.

I poured coffee into my water bottle and got on my bike. I rode directly in the middle of the four-lane road. I tried to breathe it in. I would probably never see it again like this. There was a car here and there but they seemed to have a little more respect for me, at least for my navy blue scrubs. I was essential. This was my road. I let the cars pass on the right and they never once honked at me. I guess they didn't want to ruin the calm before my storm. I got to the usually busy intersection where the train station was. I ran up the two stories, bike in hand. Very few people were around. I felt like Will Smith in "I am Legend." The scenes of an abandoned New York City, with wildlife and overgrown plant life everywhere, ran through my head, though I would have to do a lot more push-ups to look like Will in that movie. My earbuds were blasting the rest of my playlist. I boarded the empty COVID train and stared out the window of the car-connecting vestibule. We crossed the river and I followed it with my eyes, as far and as long as I could, until it was gone, then I was looking at woods and construction and new apartment complexes. My fun train ride was almost over. I rode my bike the rest of the way to work, through more empty streets, and sat down by the pond for fifteen minutes of tranquility and meditation. I thought about breathing in the fresh air and reserving that fresh air somewhere in my body, so I could draw from it while in my COVID facility, to prevent me from breathing in COVID droplets.

I got through the check-in desk at the lobby, got my double masks, and got my PPE from the improvised locker room. I went upstairs to the nursing office, and got my assignment—1A quarantine! I went to the other side of the building and back downstairs. I decided to get to the building earlier so I could actually clock in on time... not that anyone was paying particular attention to punctuality. They were lucky if anyone showed up at all.

I took report from Claudia and kicked her ass out the door. I couldn't let her get me down when I was trying to keep everyone else up. Jerard hadn't had a fever since I left him with that second dose of Tylenol last night and that news was fucking fantastic! Maybe he was coming out on the other side of the virus and on track for a full recovery. We had another two residents come to us overnight. One resident had no fever but her oxygen dipped to 91% and she complained of difficulty breathing. That was enough for a COVID admission. I felt like a game show host playing for life or death: *Well, Debbie, come on down! With your oxygen levels depleting and your lungs shutting down, you get a two-week stay on the COVID quarantine UUUUnit! At this fabulous resort, you'll have your very own nurse and CNA to check on you every couple of hours. They'll check your vital signs and give you all your medication. You won't have to see any of your family! Will you make it through? Will you succumb to this virus we call Corona!? Only time will TELLLL! Enjoy your time here on QUAAAARANTINE ISLAND!* I'm not sure why, but my mind made these types of connections and I played them out in my head. Some called it lunacy or delusional thinking—I called it in-flight entertainment. Letting my mind escape the dire situation I was in helped to relieve my stress.

My census was now eight. One of the new residents had a G-tube, so my job got a little harder. I began my med-pass very early. I didn't really care, I don't think the residents did either. I got to the G-tube resident named Mike Donald. *Two first names. I couldn't trust him.* I tried to recall G-tube administration protocols and procedures. I would have to crush up all his pills in a very fine powder. I would then mix them individually with water, then one by one, dump them into a large piston syringe temporarily connected to his G-Tube. I would then add water in between each medication. I added all the meds with my dominant right hand, all the while holding the G-tube with my pinky and ring finger and holding the piston syringe attached to it with my middle finger, index finger, and thumb... of my left hand! Dexterity was key here and I was pretty good at it—the decade of rolling joints had finally paid off. G-tube medication administration required real concentration. If you messed up here, you could spray your resident with gastric contents or mixed medications. You could spray yourself with the same and it was a common occurrence for new nurses. G-tube maintenance and medication administration was another task that made me feel like a real nurse, and not just a chump on a med-cart bargaining with the elderly to take their pills. Once you were done with the meds, you had to flush the G-Tube with the amount of water prescribed. This was for hydration for the resident as well as getting debris or remnants from the crushed medicine out of the tube, to keep it open or *patent* for the next nurse to use. If a nurse came on to the unit to see a clogged G-tube, it would ruin their day before it had even begun.

The resident with the G-tube was pretty much non-verbal. You would still explain to the resident what you were doing and why you were doing it, even if they looked like they couldn't understand or didn't talk back. It was courteous and the right thing to do. I looked for the positive things in everything. The positive thing here was that he couldn't give me any grief. He was a large man, and strong. I'd seen him in the hall all the time and remarked how large and big-boned he was, although he was not fat. Somehow I knew he would make it through his COVID sentence. I saluted him as I smiled at him and said I'd see him later. I turned around, opened the door, took my gown and gloves off as fast as possible, dumped them in the trash, stepped into the hallway, and closed the door.

I got back to my med-cart and began flipping through Mike Donald's medication records. I got to the last page to write the vital signs in. *Fuck! I forgot to take his vital signs!* I was so focused on the G-tube meds I totally forgot to see how he was doing with the virus. I probably shouldn't be a nurse. *Fuck that. I'm better than half the people here, that's why I'm in charge of these life-and-death situations after one month of experience!* My confidence came back quickly. Even if it wasn't confidence, I was the only one willing to do this job. I wasn't open to criticism at that moment nor was there anyone to critique my errors anyway. I donned my PPE again, exhaling as I did, self-pity getting the better of me. *It could always be worse.* I walked in and said hello again to Mike and told him why I was back. "I screwed up, buddy. I forgot to get your vital signs. This will only take a minute, okay?" I didn't wait for the response that would never come and placed the blood pressure cuff on his right arm. I started the machine, I found the pulse oximeter and put it on his finger. I got the temperature probe, put a plastic cover on it, and put it under his tongue. I continued to explain everything I was doing. The thermometer beeped; 97.8 degrees Fahrenheit. I look down at the pulse oximeter on his finger. 98%. The blood pressure machine beeped at the sign of completion. 132/78. His heart rate, 87. All his vital signs were fine. His breaths were even and eighteen a minute on room air. *Why was he brought down here again!?* I disconnected everything and hauled ass out of the room. As I turned around to say goodbye again, he stared at me with an empty look, but his right hand was at his forehead saluting me. I saluted him back and almost cried. Luckily there was no one on the floor to see the tears pooling in my eyes. I pulled it together and moved on. I finished the rest of my med-pass and documented some more. My shift came to an end and I relaxed at the nurse's station. I had an hour and a half to kill. I took a break while I had the opportunity.

Back at the ghost town of a nurse's station, I screwed around on my phone, checking my bank accounts and credit scores. I looked at the ESPN app but remembered nothing was happening in the world of sports. I checked Instagram for the news that the COVID was just a dream and everything would be back to normal tomorrow, but that news never came… I recounted the single narcotic and sanitized my cart. Now back on my feet, I checked on everyone once more. I debated whether or not to get some last-minute temperatures but decided against it. After all, I'd just gotten full vitals on everyone less than two hours earlier, and the oncoming nurse would no doubt do one set of vital signs early on in their shift. Besides that, these residents needed uninterrupted rest to fight the virus. I took the extra time to sanitize all the door knobs in my unit. It took less than seven minutes. In total there were close to thirty-five knobs; I thought for sure this would help flatten the curve—negative unproductive thinking got the better of me and I figured there was nothing any of us could do to flatten the curve. As I wandered the hall I wondered if there were COVID-free residents, like Jerard and Mike, and if coming down to quarantine would then subject them to the COVID when they didn't even have it to begin with. It was a terrible thought, but I had to trust that my peers, practitioners, and supervisors here would be making the right decisions… although I wasn't too confident. What if Jerard's cough was just a cough and it just happened coincidentally while COVID was beginning to take over the facility? When I thought about it, he was nowhere near resident or ground zero. Could this be a mistake? Playing out the scenario and thinking of why's and if's were going to exhaust and depress me. I needed to focus on the task at hand and the day at hand. One day at a time was my new way of life, and I made it through this day. Tomorrow would be a new day with its own challenges. Living one day at a time was the easiest way for me to live. All this other crap was out of my control and I couldn't change it so I had to accept it. I had to focus on my side of the street—or should I say my side of the facility. The COVID side.

Chapter 7

March 28th

Faith is the antidote to fear

The next day was along the same lines as the previous two on my quarantine unit. The only exception was that there were five new cases of difficulty breathing/fever/cough. Evelyn's PCR nasal swab had come back positive for the Corona Virus two days earlier. One more positive PCR result and it would be considered an outbreak. The next three residents were less than a day away from getting their results. The press was coming out with all different facts and statistics and theories. The virus could live on inanimate objects for up to three days. You could have it and not know it for seven days before symptoms set in. You could have it, have no symptoms, but still be spreading it. The press was my worst enemy at the moment. They were fear-mongering and inciting panic and mass hysteria. It sickened me. Bring us the news, but also bring us fear and intimidation. There were no puff pieces anymore, just gloom, doom, and death. They told us of a Jewish wedding in New York where there were four hundred guests. Two of them had been traveling in China. They attended the wedding, and then tested positive for the virus days after the wedding. I automatically thought, "Well, there goes the whole tristate!" Despite the grave situation all thirteen of my COVID residents faced, they were still glued to their TV sets watching ABC7 and FOX5 New York. All I heard was COVID this and COVID that. I couldn't bear it anymore! I wished I was one of those nurses with AirPods to block out the TVs, the screams, the moans, the yelling. I would never give in to this because I had to hear if someone was in trouble. I had to hear the call bell going off. Music gave me energy and would give me a smoother, faster shift, but safety was my priority and because of that I couldn't isolate myself and risk my resident's well-being. I took good care of my residents, although I missed a few sets of vitals. I had to pay particular attention to Evelyn because her oxygen had dropped to 90%. I told her to breathe deeply and put her arms up on the bedside table in front of her. I also raised the head of her bed to a 90-degree position to open her lungs up. I used all interventions and exhausted all options before deciding to put her on oxygen. I decided to make a joke about it as I placed the pulse oximeter on her finger: "90%. 90% is the final number. Do I hear 91%? Yada yada yada 91%—anyone for 91%?" I was talking fast like a southern auctioneer. I didn't know what the auctioneers said in between the numbers so I used Elaine's signature "Yada yada yada," from Seinfeld. Evelyn's eyes widened with excitement and intrigue, and she started to smile.

"Keep breathing, Evelyn!" I shot her an intense look and she followed my order. "91% Very good! Keep breathing. We got 91%! 91% going once—92%! Keep breathing! 93%. 93% can anyone do any better?" She continued to be entertained and saw that the deep breathing was working. She continued to breathe deeply. "93% going once. 93% going twice. 93% sold—94%! A new record! 94% do I hear 95%!?" If I could keep her at 94% she wouldn't need oxygen, but she probably couldn't keep up the deep breathing for too long. Even I was shocked that the deep breathing and positioning were working, and kept at it. "94% 94% yada yada yada. 94% to the women with the glasses, do I hear 95%?!" She was enjoying the personal competition of life and death, "94%,94% yada yada 94%. Do I hear 95%?! 94% going once—95%! Holy shit, Evelyn! You're doing great!"

"You watch your mouth, Mister," she said seriously, but with a smile. We were both immensely enjoying her personal triumph.

"I'm sorry Miss Evelyn! I'm just very excited! We just have to keep your oxygen up!" This little game was fun for the resident and the nurse and was one that I would revisit with other residents in other scenarios. It showed them that they might have some control over their situation and health. Evelyn was a DNR so I wouldn't have to call a code but I could tell she was still scared after all the fun and games. Not terrified, but definitely scared.

At one point, after the humor and levity left us, she realized deep breathing for the rest of her life might not be an option and asked me, "Am I going to die?" in a low, calm voice.

"Why would you say that?!" I replied in a shocked, almost offended tone. I was caught *way* off guard. I improvised well enough. They didn't tell you about this in nursing school. They said not to instill false hope or confidence, but they didn't exactly elaborate on what a proper response might be. "I'm going to take the best care of you, I promise!" *I can't promise what the next nurse will do. Here I go crying again.* My eyes were welling up as I began to plan my escape. "Just keep breathing, Evelyn! You're doing great!" (*The only thing a nurse needed in order to succeed in healthcare was a poker face*).

I went to pat her gently on the shoulder and she grabbed my hand and looked me in the eyes. "Thank you, darlin'," she said sincerely as she closed her eyes and put her head back. She believed me and she was truly grateful. I lowered the head of her bed just a little bit and told her how sitting upright while sleeping would keep her lungs open and she may have to do this for the next couple of nights. She said it was no problem. These older generations were as tough as nails and seldom scared of anything. Even with the ever-present COVID fear, Evelyn never panicked. She was a woman of great faith. "Faith is the antidote to fear, Evelyn." I felt strange trying to pep-talk a 90-year-old.

"I got plenty of that, baby. Good night." She closed her eyes again. The pulse ox was still at 95%. I figured it would drop soon, but my impeccable timing would allow me to be there just in time to administer the life-saving oxygen.

I left the pulse oximeter on her finger because I concluded that she was my most critical resident. There was one other fever on the floor—Jackson Mason. He was a younger fella who'd undergone a stroke and was left with left-sided hemiplegia. He could only use his right side but otherwise recovered well from his cerebral vascular accident. He was sixty-nine and strong. I gave him the Tylenol as needed. His fever never went beyond 101. He laughed and joked and called it the "Chinese flu," and mocked the seriousness of the virus. He said things like, "If 'Nam didn't get me, this shit ain't taking me out either!" I admired his courage and tried to carry it with me.

I went back to Evelyn. She was a fan favorite and I did not want to become known as the nurse to let her pass on to the other side. Everyone was praying for her. Everyone constantly asked me how she was doing as I came and went to my unit at the beginning and end of my shift. It was like I was her lawyer or another type of representative responsible for talking to the press on her behalf. She was like everyone's grandmother. If she liked you, she kept your important dates in her calendar. She would mark down birthdays and anniversaries of the staff and the residents, too. She also had a knack for knowing staff's children's names. I thought, if she wrote those down too, or her memory was just stellar for her age. Maybe she was a saleswoman or politician and it was just a talent that she held onto.

I checked on Evelyn again. Although my COVID roulette would be over soon and she would be the next nurse's responsibility, I wanted to do my best. Depending on what nurse walked through that door, Evelyn could be dead by the morning if no one checked on her. The pulse ox was still running and it showed 90%. I kept watching and saw it go down as low as 88% at one point and I immediately started perspiring from every pore on my body. She took a deep breath while she was sleeping and it started to climb again. Eventually, it crept up to 94%. *Thank God.*

"Keep breathing Evelyn, everyone is praying for you!" I said enthusiastically, but as quietly as possible. It was 2250 and I was ten minutes away from my relief. I gently slid off the pulse oximeter and tiptoed towards the door. I took off all my PPE and trashed it, opened the door, and quietly left. I said a prayer for her right there, outside her room. I thought that the closer I was to her, the louder God might hear the prayer, and the more inclined He would be to help.

My relief was Sarita, a Jamaican nurse and a damn good one. She was a veteran. She was truly *relief.* I knew Evelyn and all the others would be in such good hands and I could not think of a better nurse to take over. We counted the narcotics after she rounded and confirmed all thirteen souls were alive and breathing.

As I was opening the narc drawer she immediately questioned me about Evelyn. "Wah-gwon wid' Miss Evelyn? You got her on a rebreathe? What she sattin' at?"

I told Sarita her most recent oxygen saturation of 94% and how she'd been going up and down. She squeaked, put on a gown and some gloves, and entered the room. I stood and watched her. She turned the light on and put a pulse oximeter on Evelyn's finger, trying not to wake her up. She took her stethoscope and tried to auscultate Evelyn's lungs, again, trying not to wake her. Evelyn squinted her eyes open to see Sarita and smiled. "My baby, what are you doing here?!" She was excited to see Sarita.

"'Ey Mamma! 'Ow you doing?!" she enthusiastically but quietly shouted back. "Me gone take good care of ya tonight that's what, Mamma! You gone go back to bed and me see ya in da monin. Get some rest."

Evelyn obliged and went back to sleep. Sarita came out and I could tell she also got emotional. *Good thing I'm not the only one getting soft in here.*

"Oh my, me 'gone keep a tight eye on Miss Evelyn. She doin' okay right now. She gone be fine doe, she gone make it, she a strong one now."

My confidence was lifted and new life was breathed into me. I felt like I could do another eight hours, no problem.

"She a DNR now, we cooda sat 'er up and put the arms on a table but she need the sleep now, we let her rest."

I concurred and followed her back to the cart. I left the narcotic drawer open the whole time! Luckily there was no one around to steal the one bingo card full of Percocet. My CNA had already left, and the oncoming CNA was late, as per the usual. Sarita was an ass-kicker, and definitely not an ass-kisser. She was a hardworking, intelligent nurse. She did her job well, lifted up others, and taught everyone everything she knew. If she got the tiniest sense that you weren't interested in learning, she wouldn't give you another chance. You had to be like a sponge around her to absorb all the knowledge she was dropping. You could let her know you were interested in learning by only asking questions. Once she knew you wanted to learn she would tell you every step and rationale of everything she was doing, hoping you would retain 15% of what was being said. She moved quick and spoke quicker. She would throw in a question asking you to recall things from nursing school, "What you rememba' 'bout dis one 'ere?" If your mind couldn't retrieve the information fast enough, she told you the answer and kept it moving. She never made you feel bad about not knowing but insisted you be honest about things you didn't know and skills you'd never practiced before so she would know what and how to teach you. She always stood up to the doctors and administrators who would come around and try and put people in their place. She would ask them, "'Ow long you been watching this resident? Me, I been watching him five days a week fo' 'da lass tree munts!" The doctors and administrators were usually speechless and would concede. She was awesome in every single way and nurses aspired to be like her. The nurses who didn't admire or look up to her were in nursing for all the wrong reasons.

We sat and chatted after I gave her the run-down. We talked about the contagiousness of the virus. She mostly talked and I listened. She said it was too early to know anything, and as long as we kept these n95s on our faces we should be good, and I concurred. She said I did a good job with Miss Evelyn. I was enormously proud of this compliment; I wish I could have printed it out and put it on my resume. Respect from Sarita meant a great deal. And if others were around to see it, they automatically had to respect you by proxy. Unfortunately, no one witnessed the compliment, but it meant the world to me. "'Dare a reason you down here, Papa."
Because I've been a nurse for thirty-five days and won't object to a COVID assignment or cause any trouble? I blushed and gushed from the flattery all the same. I proudly told her that everyone else was fine, save for the half-ass fever Jackson Mason had. I told her the last time he had Tylenol. We said our goodbyes and good lucks. I walked out the door and onto cloud nine. Maybe the reason I was down there was because I *really* was one of the best. Hard to believe, but after getting the praise from Sarita I began to consider it as a possibility. If I had the choice I probably wouldn't have opted for the COVID unit, but I had to make the best of it. I won't ever know why I was stationed down there and I don't care. I like to think it was because of my hustle and heart, maybe not because I was the best.

I made it to the train station in what seemed like record time. The compliment was converted into energy and I pedaled fast the whole way. I enjoyed my empty train platform and let my confidence take it over. I spontaneously "whooped" and then quickly brought it back in. Up to this point in my new nursing career, there were a lot of uncertainties about my practice and what I remembered, and how I would act in certain situations. After getting a compliment from a *real* nurse you could imagine the level of excitement and pure joy I felt. I "whooped" again. My fear-driven ego told me to stop because of what others might think. *Fear.* Fear was still capable of guiding my behavior sometimes. I decided I would stop my outbursts because it was midnight and I didn't want the houses within earshot of the train station to hear me. If anyone happened to see me they would be asking themselves, "Why is this nurse so excited during a pandemic?" I got on the train and listened to my music. I'm not sure if it was the quick whoop I let out, the cold weather, or what, but suddenly I felt a tickle in my throat...

Chapter 8

March 29th

If it is thy will

I woke up with my throat aching as if I had slept in a chokehold. My sputum was yellowish/green. I had no cough, shortness of breath, or fever so I figured it was just a cold, probably from riding my bike in the frigid weather at night. I felt a little better as I drank coffee and was able to wake up, but I still decided to call out. When they asked me what my problem was, I told them sore throat and the supervisor said, "Oh… okay, I'll mark you down." I thought if I went with a "stomach bug," someone somewhere would surely say, "Oh yeah, that's been going around," and COVID wouldn't be a thought. A few months later and every symptom and sign in the book would indicate COVID, but for now it was only fever, difficulty breathing, and cough. Would my work need a sick note? A negative COVID test? Where could I get a COVID test? They still weren't available in large supplies. I called the local ER and explained the situation and that I was a nurse in a nursing home. The person (a secretary I'm guessing,) told me to come in and I could get tested.

When I arrived at the ER there was a tent outside the entrance and a nurse in full bio-hazard gear. It looked like a scene from the movie "Outbreak." She told me I wasn't guaranteed a test but I could be seen by the doctor. I explained again how I was a nurse and it was imperative that I return to work with a negative test. She stuck to the script and couldn't guarantee a test for me. She stated that they were only allotted twenty tests per day at this early stage of the pandemic. The twenty tests were reserved for the residents who exhibited symptoms of the virus and had real difficulty breathing. I got on my bike and left, angry and nervous. I waited at the bus stop on the busy main street downtown. I was the only one waiting for the bus. I waited for five minutes, caught the next bus, and headed back to my apartment. They didn't check for my fare on the bus either. I waved to Cesar from the back—I was the only one on the bus. I got home and reheated some grilled chicken. As I ate I felt every piece of food go down as if it was ping-ponging back and forth between the inflamed parts of my throat. I decided not to be seen at the ER because I had no health insurance and no assurance I could get what I needed—a COVID test. I chose to go with Urgent Care because it would be cheaper and less busy. I called the one down the street and they had no COVID tests whatsoever. I decided to go anyway because I figured I would need some type of documentation, but as I thought about it, even if I did have COVID, wouldn't I be able to work on the COVID unit? All the residents there already had it… I couldn't infect someone who was already infected. I figured the risk was in infecting people on the way to work, in and out of the non-quarantine areas at my facility.

I showed up at the Urgent Care on my bike and locked it outside. I took a minute to catch my breath. I didn't want to be breathing heavily in a packed waiting room with the pandemic approaching full swing. I wore a surgical mask and my bandana on top of it to limit exposure to civilians and non-essentials (I loved this new terminology the world was using). Luckily there were just a few people ahead of me—two fellas who looked like they were injured on the job. I wondered what they did for work during the shutdown—maybe they were stock boys in a supermarket—it was the only job I could think of at that moment that might still be operating. I was called in less than a half-hour. The medical assistant took my vital signs and left. The doctor saw me five minutes after that. The doctor was a middle-eastern woman, who also happened to be pregnant. She was wearing full PPE with n95 and surgical masks but I still blurted out that my condition might be COVID and I had been working on a COVID unit the last week. She showed no fear and looked in my throat. She ordered a rapid strep test. I thought about the doctor and her dauntless approach… Candace had gotten into a car accident a month before and spoke about this doctor and how wonderful and pregnant she was. She looked like she could give birth any second. I was confident I could deliver her baby if God willed it…as I began to digress to scenes of my triumphant and miraculous delivery she came back less than five minutes later and said "Yup! Its strep! Have you ever had strep throat before?"

I told her how I'd had it once or twice as a kid. She wrote the script for the antibiotics and I was on my way, but not before I got my 'return to work' note. She gave me three days in addition to that day I was seen by her in the urgent care.

I got home and remarked on Instagram how delighted and excited I was for the diagnosis to be strep throat and not a *deadly* COVID one. Anyone would take a diagnosis of strep throat these days over the dreaded COVID. I also took the time to write a five-star Yelp review for the urgent care and mentioned the doctor's name for her expedient and thorough care. I believed in good reviews and bad ones. For every bad review I left, I made sure to balance the world's energy with a good one. I told Candace the news and she was relieved. Candace half-heartedly volunteered to drive me to the pharmacy but I knew she'd feel uncomfortable in close proximity to me in the car. Her proposition was empty but I appreciated the gesture anyway. I road a couple of blocks on the mostly empty streets to the pharmacy where I could pick up my Azithromycin. I waited at the pharmacy longer than at the urgent care—at least it seemed like it. While I waited I gave the urgent care another five-star review, on Google this time. I felt inclined to do so, as I compared the two wait times. I didn't have anything to do the rest of the day. No gym. No meetings. No work. Maybe just a Tiger King marathon.

I got back around three o'clock in the afternoon. I would just be starting work on the COVID unit at this time if I'd been feeling healthy. I wondered how many more souls had been sentenced to a two-week quarantine. I wondered how many PCR tests had come back positive. How many were negative. I prayed for their health and safety. I prayed for the staff I left behind for the King of tigers. I did some push-ups and sit-ups before we started the binge of the King. We had a handful of episodes left. I planned to do more push-ups and sit-ups in between them all. Gym and exercise were a huge part of my sobriety. They gave me a healthy high and kept "stinking thinking" at bay. I always told people how working out kept me in a good mood. I never had to deal with real depression before but I know that for me, exercise kept me from feeling sad.

We watched three episodes back to back. I didn't do any exercises between the episodes like I thought I would. We took a break from the couch and I took the opportunity to bang out a hundred of each. I meandered around the apartment and looked out the front windows to see a homeless crackhead sitting outside the 7-11 asking for money. He had no shirt on and no mask. It was warmer and he was right in the sun but he had to have been cold unless the drugs he was on were keeping him warm. People walking past him would step into the parking lot from the sidewalk in an attempt to keep six feet from him. Maybe he hadn't caught the news—he probably didn't even have a living room to have a TV in. I felt bad for him but didn't pray for him at that moment. I made my bed and read the day's Daily Interpretations. Daily Interpretations was a book from my Alcohol Support Group's global literature department. It had 365 days of personal anecdotes, stories, and prayers to help keep the sober alcoholic on the straight and narrow. After reading the day's message, I prayed for the homeless man with no shirt. I did a couple more sets of push-ups and sit-ups as fast as I could, hoping to get a cardiovascular pump in the process. It got me sweaty and I showered. I wasn't hungry yet so we decided to keep watching the King.

After watching one more episode we decided to take a walk and get some fresh air before dinner. There was no one outside except for a few people coming and going at the 7-11. The homeless man must have begged enough money to get his next fix and find an alley to sleep in. I prayed for him again. I wore a mask only because I knew I had an infection and I could spread it just by breathing if by chance passing another person on my walk. We walked along Lonzo Avenue for blocks and blocks. Everything was very surreal. We passed a normally busy and happening church. Its parking lot was empty, as was the inside. Normally you could peek through the windows to see members of the congregation busy with choir practice, arts and crafts, and volunteer work. Now, there was only darkness, except for the glowing lettering of an exit sign towards the back of the church. I asked myself how the congregation would get their spiritual refreshment. Perhaps the pastor or reverend was tech-savvy and had his flock on Zoom already. I decided to visit the church for Mass once it reopened. I made a plan to make a large donation to help keep the lights on so I didn't have to see the sad and meek EXIT sign through the dark chapel.

We came back through the dark and empty waiting room and climbed the stairs. I passed the laundry and made a mental note that I would do the washing tomorrow on my unplanned day off. I had an appetite now and cooked some chicken stir-fry. Peppers, onions, broccoli, and cubed pieces of chicken. The whole apartment heated up instantly. I thought it might be good for my ear, nose, and throat to breathe in steamed air, but we had to open all the windows to cool the apartment. As I smelled the food I got hungrier and hungrier. I recapped the day and figured I'd expended a lot of energy biking all around the city, doing my exercises, and stressing. I was definitely in a caloric deficit for the day. I thought of my coworkers and my residents. I thought of Evelyn and whether or not I could grace her with my presence again, or she mine. I prayed for her and asked God to pull her through… if it was His will—when it came to my prayers, I felt odd telling God what to do and whom to help, and what to give them. I could only hope that He heard my prayers and considered them. I ended every prayer with, "If it is thy will," to make sure I wasn't pissing Him off. I thought of calling the facility for updates but figured I didn't want to bother the already taxed and tired nurses.

I filled my plate with my stir-fry. I was impressed with the outcome. I got a seltzer, grabbed the remote, resumed the show, and sat down. The Tiger man was *threatening* some woman for *threatening his* business. I felt sad for both of them. When movies or TV got to the sad parts, to make myself better I would always say, "It's okay, don't be sad. This isn't real." I couldn't use this platitude for The Tiger King documentary because it was actually a true story. Their situation had really gotten out of hand. I got a kick out of it until my grim outlook on society got the better of me…

We had one episode left and decided to save it for the next morning—I needed to do something for my sobriety. By this time, all Alcohol Support Group meetings in my area had been closed down for a couple of weeks now, just like everything else. Since the Alcohol Support Group meetings were suspended, they took to Zoom and were absolutely flourishing and thriving in their new online home. There were meetings all day long from all over the world. It was an incredibly fast mobilization. All the donations that members had previously made to their in-person meetings would go to the global fund, and now to Zoom, for the required hour-long subscriptions. Alcohol Support Group and Zoom enabled all the alcoholics and addicts in the world to get the fellowship and support they needed to stay sober. Some of the larger local meetings continued their meetings online. New local online meetings popped up. Mega meetings with hundreds of people became a norm. I preferred the mega meetings because it was with people I had never seen before and stories I'd never heard, from places I'd never been. The one meeting was the Twenty-four-Hour Marathon Meeting. This meeting had been running literally non-stop since mid-March. How long could the marathon meeting last?! This required tons of organization and volunteers doing service work. One would be the greeter, one would be the chair, one would be the treasurer with a couple of other co-hosts—but that was only for one hour! They then had to fill this number of positions for the other twenty-three hours in a day, then keep it going seven days a week for the next year or more! It was incredible what we were doing to stay sober and to help others do the same.

I joined one of the local meetings that took to the airwaves and said hello to all of my friends. Some of the older members weren't exactly the best with technology, especially when it came to microphones, cameras, and live web streaming. It was funny to watch them fiddle and struggle with the new norm. Eventually, it became irritating when they couldn't mute their mic and we heard their obnoxious breathing or their cat or bird that wouldn't shut up. It took another week or two before all of the hosts knew how to find and mute the audio offenders. It had its negatives and positives but it was *most certainly* better than no meetings at all. Only a couple of weeks in and the Zoom meetings began to require passwords. Apparently, there were Zoom-Bombers attending meetings for their entertainment and amusement. I heard a story from a friend that there were men in woman's only meetings asking them to "show their tits." Leave it to the bad apples in the world to try and sabotage the good folk trying to stay sober! *How dare they!*

I finished my meeting, said good night, and got into some ice cream thinking it might soothe my sore throat. I took my antibiotics with water while digging into some "Tonight Dough" from my friends, Ben and Jerry. I only ate ice cream once every two weeks on my weekend off. I figured since I was sick, it was a good occasion to break my twice-monthly ice cream allotment. Looking at the antibiotics, I feared I would forget to take them. I was never good with reminders and to-do lists, so I figured I would leave sticky notes around my apartment regarding my meds. I didn't want to miss any doses for fear of the bug becoming resistant. I settled for one sticky note in the bathroom where I would see it a dozen times a day. There was no way I could forget now.

The next day was more of the same, my throat wasn't improving. Candace and I watched Netflix, I worked out and listened to music, and then we walked about a mile. I had nowhere to go by bike so I didn't ride at all. Biking was solely transportation; I didn't take leisure rides. The rest of the country was getting into outdoor activities, especially biking. I didn't see an influx of riders around me but heard about bike shops being sold out. I figured the next time I was in the area I would check out the bike shop where I bought mine. I had to see if the biking movement had really taken off in my area. I was happy for people getting more exercise and time with the family... while getting paid for it! People were starting to get unemployment and talks of stimulus packages and additional unemployment were becoming very popular. Only in America, baby!

I attended two online meetings. One of the speakers spoke about being at the bar with friends, pulling down his pants zipper, and urinating right where he sat. He wasn't black-out drunk but he said he didn't care at the time. I could relate to the story. I'd never done this but I'm sure I'd done equally offensive acts. Once I popped that first beer, I couldn't stop. Thinking back on my lifestyle and the decade-plus of drinking every day always made me cringe. I would try to stop thinking about those things and to thank God that today I was sober and I had a new life for myself. After the meetings, I called some sober alcoholics in my network. I caught up with the ones who took my call and left funny messages for the ones who didn't. In my area's meetings, I was known for phoning newcomers, and freestyle rapping for them on their voicemail when they didn't pick up. I just wanted to reach out and let them know life after alcohol didn't have to be so serious or dull. I talked to Bret who was actually from Wisconsin, and decided to grace him with some freestyle sobriety rap:

Hey Yo Brett! what's going on,
You didn't pick up so, I'm gonna sing this song,

If I was still drinking I'd be long gone,
Drunken stupor and black-out wasted,
But sobriety is the best thing I ever tasted
I'll probably never meet you,
But if I did I would surely greet you,
Keep it up one day at a time and don't slack
And no matter what, keep coming back!

Then I would tell him what Zoom meeting I met him in and tell him I could relate to his twenty-seven days sober, and how it felt and how it keeps getting better. Some would call back and others wouldn't. I did it to make newcomers feel welcome and liked, and to show them that phoning a friend didn't have to be an hour long heart-to-heart, but more of a check-in. These phone calls helped me stay happy and sober. In order to maintain our sobriety we had to help others to do the same—we had to give away what was so freely given to us and I chose to do it light-heartedly and comically. Sobriety was our priority but we sober alcoholics were capable of living full and fun lives. My new lot of friends were anything but glum.

I went to bed, got up the next morning, and did it all again. I would return to work the following day to see how COVID was treating my facility. I figured there would be more cases. I figured I'd be back down on quarantine. I figured I would get some type of good news; for there had been nothing but bad news the last three weeks. Tides would turn for sure.

Chapter 9

April 3rd

After perfecting the poker face, the nurse must learn to walk, talk and think like a detective. Through this skill, the nurse will gain knowledge and information others might have overlooked.

My return to work was easy. After the thermo-gun, the sign-in, and the makeshift PPE locker room in the conference room, I proudly presented my sick note from the urgent care to the scheduler and payroll person, Carrie. The sick note meant I was being honest and I didn't call out to go to a three-day music festival or to nurse a hangover. In the past, I used sick time for such reasons. I was used to being dishonest and I always feared getting caught, but I didn't have to think like this anymore. I was expecting some type of reaction or relief from her, but she just took it in her hand and placed it to the side. I asked for it back and made a copy so I would have it for my records. I could see that the note getting lost in her pile of papers on her desk was a possibility and a probability. I gave it back to her and said thank you. I turned and walked out. She was clearly preoccupied with staffing a whole facility during a pandemic—I couldn't blame her. I was shocked when I got my assignment of 2B—my home. I thought to myself that I should be on 1A with my quarantine COVID buddies since I had started out with them. I immediately started questioning who was down there, and why. Were they better than me? Did someone volunteer? Maybe they just forgot I'd been stationed down there for three days. I turned off my speculative thinking and got to work. *Don't think—just do.*

Walking down the long hall was like walking through a busy Diagon

Alley, except there were no wizards, just people in blue gowns, surgical caps, face masks, and goggles. Some people I could recognize by the eyes, others I had no clue about, but I tried to say hello to everyone regardless. As I approached 2B, I found an agency nurse at my desk and not Tanya. She was covered in plastic and wore her surgical mask over her n95. She wore a face shield and a surgeon's cap over her head. The only human parts I could see were her eyes. I walked past the nursing station and said, "Hey I'm your relief—how are you?" in a solemn tone.

"I'm good, thanks," she barely looked up and returned to what she was doing.

I kept walking and decided to round on all my residents like a good nurse. This was a fundamental, and these types of fundamentals saved lives and licenses. Fundamentals and basics were also important in recovery. I had to keep doing the things that got me sober and I had to do all the nursing fundamentals to keep people healthy—or, during a pandemic—*alive*.

I worried about some more than others. In the corner with the quadruple rooms and the utility room, I saw that Wally Lasiter was missing. I made a mental note of it and continued my tour. Barbara Watkins was also gone. I started to panic… Belle Montagne's room was vacant as well. Everyone else was there. Three of my regular twenty-seven residents were missing. They couldn't be at a doctor's appointment. They couldn't be at a recreation event. They couldn't be in the dining room. All these activities had been canceled because of the COVID. I went to get my report from the space lady. She gave a quick report and mentioned how at the moment there were no fevers. We counted the narcotics quickly. I saved my questions and let her leave. The priority at this time was to monitor the residents I *did* have and check their vital signs. At the first sign of fever or difficulty breathing, I would report my findings to management and await orders to quarantine. I still didn't know where my three residents were, but I knew more would be revealed in time. I figured this agency nurse, whose name I never got, was only working today and didn't even have the answers as to where those residents had gone. For all she knew, they had never even been there. *They probably went viral.*

I checked their MAR and saw that all three resident's records were not in there. They must have been sent to quarantine. I focused on the task at hand. I focused on what I could control and who I could take care of. After organizing and cleaning the desk (something the previous nurse didn't do), I checked my med-cart for silly stock meds to make sure they were full. I walked around and took a couple of vital signs of residents who were willing and not busy with something else.

I got back to my desk around 1600 to find the supervisor waiting for me. It was Sarita! Our fearless leader. She usually didn't supervise so I assumed we were short-staffed, and she'd gotten the call up to the majors.

She was sitting at my clean and organized desk, working on her clipboard. She looked up, and started filling in, "'Ey, 'ow you doing, Papa? We 'eard ya got da COVID now? Why ya back so soon?!" She didn't wait for me to answer. "So, you seen ya got tree residents down on da quarantine? Wally, Barbara, and Belle all down dare 'anging out wit miss Claudia, 'dey 'avin a grand ole' time all locked up an' down." She chuckled and continued, "Tanya out with fever and cough, we think it's COVID. She gone get tested today or tomorrow. Gotta find a place to do 'dat for 'er."

Yea, tell me about it! I went through the same bullshit three days ago! I wanted to scream. *If everyone is worried about the elderly in nursing homes, why can't the staff taking care of said elderly get tested when they suspect COVID?!* "Okay, okay, when did Tanya go out?" I replied, knowing that her time was precious and that she moved quickly. She'd already gotten up from the chair and made for the long corridor back to the center of the building when she chose to begrudgingly respond to my question. I thought that was funny.

"Two day ago. No. Tree. I don't know, she not 'ere baby, all they need is you, Papa." And she was gone. Halfway down the hall, her walk became a slow-paced run.

Knowing that I had a real nurse at the helm gave me confidence and relief. If I had to call on her, she'd come and help, but I had to make sure I had all my boxes checked and I wasn't missing anything when I did. Otherwise, I would upset her and embarrass myself. If I made mistakes and missed things and then called Sarita, she would find the supply I was missing or the piece of information I'd overlooked, and blow me up in a funny obnoxious way for all to hear. I didn't mind, and it made me a better nurse. There was a difference between nurses totally reaming someone out and being an asshole about it, and the way Sarita did it. She made sure you got the point, but you could laugh it off and move on. No one's ego was damaged too badly when Sarita was around and teaching. For instance, if we missed a basic skill or fact about nursing, she would say something like, "Oh, you was absent."

"Wait, what?" The nurse would stutter confusingly.

"'Dat day when 'day taught you 'bout insulin prep in nursing school, you wasn't 'dare dat day, eh?" She would elaborate while smiling.

I continued to try to be the champion Sarita was. In certain situations, I would ask, *"What would Sarita do?"*

I started on my vital signs since it was a little too early for medications. I got six sets of vital signs done and had eighteen more to do. Then I would have to get all the vital signs *again* during the second half of the shift! All this, plus giving two med-passes… the task was daunting, so I thought of my mother's wisdom this time; "How do you eat an elephant? One bite at a time."

I got to work and started to wonder if anyone in the world eats elephants. *They're probably endangered. What would they taste like?* I concluded that they were just too damn majestic to be part of anyone's cuisine.

I started with the scream queens in the quadruple room. Jan Konkle and Leanne Donovan. As I donned my PPE from their doorway I observed their behavior. I heard them before I could even see them. They were in rare form, screaming obscenities. Usually, when they were especially loud and vulgar like this, it meant some type of care hadn't been given to them. Although their conscious minds were all but gone, their bodies felt when they were deprived of something or they weren't being taken care of. The brain-speech connection still worked for them and they would let everyone know it, although the content of their hysterical obscene rants was non-sensical. I still felt bad for them, regardless of the grief they caused everyone. I put on my detective hat and started the investigation. There was no water at either bedside. They could be dehydrated. I checked the brief of one of them and found that it was wet. Dehydrated—check. Sitting in their own waste—check. I couldn't check off hunger because there were no trays in the room to see how much or how little they had eaten. The lunch trays would have been cleared out three hours ago, but it *was* a possibility that no one had set them up to eat. I also couldn't rule out that their medication was given to them. Most nurses who didn't know the two screamers, would turn right around and walk out at the first sign of trouble. I decided I would change the brief. Since I wasn't fully prepared when starting the task, it took me about twelve minutes when it should have taken me five. I had to run in and out getting extra gloves, finding linens and briefs, and changing my PPE each time I did. It wasn't my job but I couldn't leave her like that. They were yelling the whole time I was in there, and by the time I exited the room, my scrub top was completely saturated with sweat. It was an unusually warm April day and the AC units had not been turned on this early in the season. Couple this with the fact we were on the second floor made it even hotter, plus all the plastic PPE we were wearing prohibited proper ventilation. I felt disgusting already and I still had seven and a half hours to work! The game show host screamed in my head: *Winner Winner! Nursing home dinner!*

I took a deep breath, exhaled, exited the room, put on new PPE, and went into the next. Frank Dusen was sleeping soundly. COVID couldn't bother this tough fisherman… yet. It was certainly in the room if Wally Lasiter had signs and symptoms… it was only a matter of time before it reached six feet over to Frank. Jim Moss was also resting, but he always sensed when someone was entering the room, even if you were being quiet as a mouse. He still wouldn't talk too much to me. Just yes and no answers. Both their temperatures were good and their other vital signs were within normal limits. I gave them their medicine and exited the room.

Still sweating, I ran to the bathroom and relieved myself. I probably drink about forty ounces of diluted black coffee and another gallon-and-a-half of water each day. A third of this total amount is consumed before I arrive at work each day. I am constantly running to the bathroom to relieve myself. I wet my forehead with the wet paper towel I used to dry my hands and it provided momentary comfort. I blasted out of the bathroom, got back to my med-cart, and put some new PPE on, to find Tabatha Patterson freaking out. She tried to fill me in on the welfare of the floor; she did it slowly and painfully. It felt like she averaged five words per minute. She was eighty-nine, though. She'd turn ninety over the summer… if she was able to evade the omnipresent COVID. Surely she would become another nursing home statistic if she ever got it…

Anyway, I put on my poker face and pretended to listen, feigning interest. She didn't have much of a social life at this juncture in her life, so interacting with the staff was very important. Her roommate Ruby was not one for conversation and if she did feel like talking it was probably in German. I looked up the word for *friend* in German and paired it with my already acquired knowledge of *guten tag* and would tell her, "Guten tag mein freundin!"

Ruby would say, "Oh ya ya, guten tag!" And then start to speak some other German, and I'd let her. When I was done with Ruby I would say, "Auf wiedersehen!" and she would say the same back.

Once I was done with the two I turned back to Tabatha, "Thanks for the update Tabatha, you need anything else?" I immediately regretted asking that second part. *I don't want to de-gown, go out, re-gown to come back in. Shit!*

"I… need… water," she said to me slowly.

"Ok! Give me a little bit!" I said as I walked out, eyes wide with anger, silently shouting the words "*fuck me*" under my double masks. I always asked if someone needed anything on my way out, but with the workload in front of me, I realized I might have to skip that part of the routine. Some residents had nothing important for me to do but would literally look around the room and find some busy work for me to do. *Not during this fucking pandemic, damn it!* I should be grateful for Tabatha's thirst because most of my elderly residents didn't want to drink any water at all, which presented a myriad of problems for the nurse.

Luckily as I came out, I saw my CNA, Sunny, at the hot corner. I yelled, "Thank God it's Sunny!" It was a true praise of gratitude to God. When Sunny was around, the nurse had so much less to worry about. You knew that every resident would get changed as many times as they needed. You knew Sunny would never give you lip, and she'd even look out for other things that other CNAs didn't have the wit or desire to help the nurse with. Sunny was getting "PPE ready" to go see Tabatha and Ruby Vedder. I told her to wait while I got water for her to bring in. This type of teamwork and coordination would limit risk of exposure. We had to time things and make the most out of each PPE-filled journey into each room. I came back and handed it to Sunny the astronaut, thanking her for saving me that extra trip, the extra time, the extra work, and possibly the extra exposure to the COVID.

I moved to Leslie Dawson, and Barbara Watkins—shoot—now on

quarantine! Poor thing. There was no doubt she could handle loneliness and isolation, but I wasn't too confident her old and feeble body could combat the COVID effectively. She also wouldn't be getting much care down there. The nurses and CNAs had to limit *their* exposure as well, and it was more important in quarantine that they did because they were dealing with the real and contagious cases of the virus. Up here, exposure to the virus was possible but not confirmed since none of the residents showed signs or symptoms. I pondered how many more positive PCR tests came back… I opted not to pray at that moment, thinking of Evelyn and my other buddies down there. I don't know why I didn't pray. Did I not have the time?

Leslie was also sitting in a wet diaper. I gave the CNAs the benefit of the doubt and figured she had just gone. Since Sunny was around I could briefly mention a brief change and it would be done yesterday. I didn't have time to change the brief anyway. I still needed fifteen more sets of vitals signs, plus the 1700 med-pass, plus auscultating (listening through a stethoscope) forty-eight lungs belonging to twenty-four residents. The problem with listening to lung sounds was it required the nurse to be in the immediate airspace of the resident. A standard stethoscope was usually about twenty-two inches long. Even at the maximum distance, you were still less than two feet from the air the residents were breathing in and out. You had to make sure none of your mucous membranes were exposed to air or else any COVID particles lurking could find their way into your respiratory tract.

After Leslie's lonely room, I went to Lucie Greer and Julie Walton and concluded that they were safe. Their vital signs were within normal limits and their lung sounds, I concluded, were clear. I came out to find the nursing supervisor Sarita waiting for me at my cart, scribbling on her clipboard. She looked up at me and I knew it wasn't good news.

"Davey, mah boy, me got some bad news 'ere."

"Aw man—who died?" I asked, more concerned than anything, but knowing Sarita would find this comic relief funny. People always said this when entering a room that wasn't exactly bubbling with enthusiasm. With COVID, death was always near and always imminent every day. So that question could have been answered that day, by Sarita telling me a gentleman from the other side of the second floor passed away early in the morning. I waited a fraction of a second for her news but it seemed like an eternity.

"We ain't got a nurse on BC side so you'll have to split the cart with Gabby." She gave me no time to object, "She already counted the cart and got report on all the residents," she turned and walked away.

I just said, "Okay." She apologized and walked off. *Fuck!* I had heard of nurse call-outs and understaffing, forcing this assignment-and-a-half on a nurse but hadn't experienced it yet. Now I had to do it with full PPE in and out of each room, two sets of vitals on each resident, *and* I had to do so on two med-carts. We would also have to coordinate when we could share the cart. I had to take my supplies to the other cart and work there while leaving my residents on my side completely alone. This was a mess. What could I say? I couldn't do anything but my best. I was immediately in a sour mood. I had to be short and to the point with each and every resident. After taking on another thirteen residents there was really no time for chit-chat. No time for cleaning up the rooms. No time for the extras. I was crying inside. I realized there would be no help coming for me or Gabby; I felt like we were the last ones on the island after the rest of the castaways were airlifted out…we could only wave goodbye at the helicopter.

I ran to the bathroom and said the Serenity Prayer while relieving myself and again while I washed my hands. I figured if I hurried up and finished my med-pass by 1730 before dinner came, I could bang out a couple on the BC side before everyone ate. Before my plan would come to fruition I had to drop what I was doing and help Jared Bartell, who was a BC resident. He was a VIP—Very *Imresident* Person. He wanted all this meds right at 1700. I was already late.

He found me down the hall. "Hey Dave? You my nurse, right? I'm ready."

I wanted to yell at him with all the fury building inside, *Well, I'm busy so I'll let you know when I'M READY! And you're not supposed to be out of your room, you piece of shit!* All I squeezed out was, "Be right there, Jared." He did whatever he wanted whenever he wanted and when you tried to ask him to obey the rules he threatened you with violence (The things nurses put up with!).

I was muttering to myself as I walked the length of my forty-yard hallway and half of the hundred-yard hallway. Gabby was on the cart so I had to wait until she was in the room giving the medications she'd just prepared. I flipped the MAR to Jared's records and prepared his medication. He was a blood sugar and blood pressure check. I looked for the glucometer and it was nowhere to be found. I could either wait till Gabby came out of the room to ask her if she knew where it was, or run back 150 yards to get my glucometer. I chose to get my own supplies because there was a good chance Gabby didn't know where it was. From my brief and limited experience and observations of her, she was never organized and always behind. I brought all the medications I had just prepared with me back the 150 yards to my med-cart—I didn't want Gabby mistaking them for hers. I gathered my glucometer, lancets, glucometer strips, and alcohol swabs, as well as my vital sign machine/rolling cart. I went right to Jared's. I started his blood pressure, and as the cuff on his arm started to inflate I took his blood sugar on his middle finger on the opposite arm. It read 228. He would get sliding-scale coverage of 6 units, plus 10 units standing dose before dinner. He also demanded we give him his 56 units of long-lasting insulin that were due at 2100, right now. I gave him two injections, watched him take his meds, and got the hell out of Dodge. He was trying to talk to me, but I just attempted to *yes* him to death. A series of uh-huhs and yeah, I knows, let him know I was listening and not ignoring him. If I ignored him completely he would threaten to "beat my ass." He knew I was busy and knew I was in no mood to hang around and shoot the shit. He was one of those people you just kept happy to avoid confrontations—in Jared's case, physical ones. He had been in the facility for over ten years so when nurses were short he recognized the extra work the nurses undertook, but didn't care. He was always "helping" staff and other residents, but with every seemingly good deed, you would have to look beyond it to find his secret motive. Detectives again. If he was pushing the dinner cart, he was quietly looking for alcohol Sani naps that he could consume in hopes to get a drunk. He was also stealing the entire pack of cookies at the bottom of that same dinner cart which was intended for everyone, which was the reason he needed the 70-plus units of insulin. I was thinking what a piece of shit he was but tried not to judge. Life must suck in a nursing home for someone who is completely sound of mind and body, especially during this pandemic.

I arrived back at my med-cart to find it completely unlocked. This wasn't the first time I left it unlocked and stepped away for a long period of time…*I gotta stop doing that!* No one was around to steal medications and narcotics but my mistake still thrust me into a rage of self-pity—*Well, if we had proper staffing I wouldn't be making errors. Shame on them for forcing this insurmountable task on me! It's not my fault, I'm the victim.* The more adversity I was facing the shittier my thinking got. I took some breaths and said the Serenity Prayer *again* as I opened the drawers of the cart. Saying my prayers always helped me. After feeling a little better I completed the 1700 med-pass for my twenty-four original residents.

I went to the other cart halfway down the hundred-yard football hallway and coordinated some more with Gabby to try and do the residents as best we could without getting in each other's way. I had two residents with gastrostomy tubes. I found that one of them was clogged and nothing would pass through it. It took ten minutes to unclog it. At first, I tried the soap trick. I put soap on my hands and milked the tube, feeling for a clog and trying to dislodge it. Once that didn't work I had to get a disposable plastic instrument that was basically a long, thin pipe cleaner. I pushed and pulled back and forth, trying to clean the inner tube. After thoroughly cleaning the inside it finally took water. I gave the resident his medications and then flushed the tube with water to make sure nothing would build up while he got his 1200 ml of liquid nutrition over the next fourteen hours. The resident kept asking me what was the matter and why I was huffing and puffing. I briefly described what I was going through and he said to me in a low, quiet voice, "Come on man, it can't be that bad. Hang in there."

Holy shit! That's my line! I laughed in my head and took it as a sign. I guess it wasn't that bad, I just kept doing the best I could.

I gave report around 0030 (a whole hour late). My thirty-seven residents—yes—thirty-seven—and all their vital signs kept me an hour and a half late. The oncoming nurse was an agency one that I had never met. She sat at the desk on her phone until I was ready for her. She arrived half an hour late anyway, so I wasn't worried. She looked like she wasn't really interested—who would be? It was her first day at the facility and I tried to fill her in and give her a decent report. No residents were going out and no doctors were coming in so there weren't any new orders to relay. I did mention the vital signs twice a shift and she laughed. "Yeah, that's not happening; I'll do my best though!" she said sarcastically with a thumbs up in my direction.

I started to worry for this nurse I had never met before. *What? But you have to! It's an order! They'll catch you and write you up! They'll fire you and take your license!* I didn't say anything except, "Yup, do what you want." I was worried I came off rude.

After we counted the narcs, she sat back down and got on her phone. I sat beside her for another half-hour charting on certain residents who needed it. I also had to sign my treatment book. *Fuck! My treatment book!* I didn't do any treatments on any of my residents or the refugee residents from 2BC. I really felt like crying at that moment. This would take me another hour at least. I got the treatment book out and skimmed through it. I found two treatments in addition to the one I knew I had to do for Adrian Larson. I would have to wake these residents up—they were no doubt sleeping at 0100 in the morning. Adrian was in a constant cycle of sleeping and coming to. He was especially combative when I told him of my intent to turn him and clean him and stick some new medicated gauze in his rear.

"You fuck!" were his first words to me during this encounter. He closed one eye and focused on me with the good eye.

I exhaled and laughed, "Come on, Adrian, I know it's late but we gotta take care of your wound."

"Leave my buddy alone!" Wally Lasiter spoke up from the next bed.

I started laughing out loud because it was too funny not to. *Everyone was up!* All the physical exhaustion and mental stress left my body in that instant and I enjoyed the moment. It was also special when I saw residents sticking up for other residents. It made me happy. I believe helping others is an innate trait of human nature, although there are certainly exceptions. Adrian was about to go in on another tirade when I saw the cases of soda on the floor next to him. "How about a soda, Adrian?" I could see his previous thoughts were abandoned and his face turned to a hopeful one.

"Okay asshole, but get some ice."

"No problem buddy, stand by." I took his cup, left the room, doffed the PPE, and found the ice chest completely empty. I huffed and puffed all the way down the football hallway to the 2C kitchenette. I blasted the cup with some ice and walked the hundred-yard football hallway back. I put the cup down outside the door as I donned a new set of PPE. I entered, found the root beer at the bedside, and poured it over the ice. It looked and sounded particularly tantalizing. I contemplated stealing a can for myself while he was sleeping but decided against it. He took a sip and sighed, and I laughed. It was like he'd cracked a beer after a long day's work. This did the trick because he even turned on his side all by himself.

"Okay come on! Come on!"

I was taken off guard—I hadn't even prepped my *procedure* table. I hurried the best I could. I pulled out old bloody gauze and started cleaning. This apparently was too long for Adrian to be on his side, or maybe he just didn't like me, but he rolled back on his butt and said, "Soda!"

I brought the soda to his mouth and let him drink.

He finished his sips and sighed. Somehow he knew we weren't done because he rolled over on his side again and said more calmly, "Okay, come on."

Note to self: bribe the resident with soda and offer sips in-between steps of the treatment. I would have to share this with other nurses. Maybe they already knew this trick but chose not to enlighten me—*no way, this wound just isn't improving, nobody gives a shit.* I finished the treatment and got the hell out of there.

After this enormous triumph, I got a second wind and finished the other two treatments which were anti-fungal creams. My night was done— oh wait!—I had to go back to 2BC to see what *other* treatments fate had in store for me. I had to do one more wound treatment and several other lotions, ointments, and creams. The 2BC assignment had a lot of bed-ridden people, people who couldn't turn themselves or care for themselves at all, so their skin had a lot more tending to than my side. I was dead tired and decided to only do the one wound treatment that I actually found. The customer was easy enough and I was in and out, wasting more plastic as I did.

I returned to my desk, gathered my things, cleaned them with bleach, put them in my backpack, and left. I was walking down the hundred-yard football hallway thinking I couldn't do too much of this thirty-seven resident stuff. But, unfortunately for me and all the other nurses, this would become the norm. I walked out of the building at about 0200 in the morning. Two and a half hours late.

Chapter 10

April 4th

God never gives you anything you can't handle

Because of my late departure the night before, I'd missed my train and had to ride the empty streets an extra three miles, bringing my total for the day to seven miles. I also racked up three hours of overtime, which I was happy about. I didn't get to bed until 4 a.m. I slept till 1:30 p.m. I was completely drained. I was physically and emotionally exhausted. This should have been my day off but they called and asked me to come in. I wasn't doing anything so I told them I would. Candace wasn't particularly happy with my decision to help but I knew the facility needed employees to pick up shifts. I weighed Candace's unhappiness with the prospect of overtime and helping the declining residents and decided that working was the right choice. I also considered that too much time at home with Candace wouldn't be good either. She'd already had cabin fever for weeks, and every time we were in the apartment it seemed like she was freaking out about something—cleaning the apartment, cleaning the groceries, waiting for her unemployment to come through, or when all of it will be over. I couldn't make her see my way or use my reasoning. "One day at a time" didn't work for her, nor did "It could always be worse." These mottos and credos seldom work on non-addict/alcoholics. She was beginning to unravel and every time I offered a different perspective she just became angry with me.

Prayer was the only part of my daily routine that I was able to do that day. I couldn't work out, I couldn't make it to an online Alcohol Support

Group meeting. I made eggs, got dressed and hurried past Candace, and past the garbage bag at the bottom of the stairs. I locked my apartment door and locked the waiting room door. *Shit!* I left my headphones in my apartment. I remembered they had come out of my bag when I had pulled my phone out the night before. I forgot to put them back in. I would have to ride in silence. Normally I could hear the hustle and bustle of the streets, but there were only so many cars back on the road. I did see a family gathering at one of the houses and they did not care at all about social distancing and only half of them were wearing masks.

I got to work and completed all my check-ins and wardrobe changes. I got to the nursing office and confirmed that I was stationed on my 2B home. I also got half of 2BC again. The game show played in my head, *"Well, David, if twenty-four residents weren't enough, we have a wonderful surprise for you! Twelve more residents are stationed far, far away from your 2B unit! Enjoy the long corridor of residents with diabetes, heart failure, and hyperrrrr-tension! And if anyone dies or gets hurt, we'll come to you and take yourrr nursing license! Enjoy the COVID Wheel of Misfortune!"*

FUCK! FUCK! FUCK! How could I be expected to do this again?! Don't they know I'm a new nurse!? No one's going to help me!? Put me back down on the COVID unit! At least I would have less residents there! I came in on my day off for this shit!? My mind was racing as I slowly walked out. My day was already ruined and it hadn't even begun. I thought of a different way to look at this quagmire and came up with the following: *If I didn't come in, that would leave one nurse for seventy-plus residents.* I thought of the lone nurse and decided my selfless thinking was noble. Then it all turned to rage again. It festered in my head as I walked down the football hallway to my hot corner which was still ice cold.

I got report and counted drugs. I didn't know who I was relieving and didn't care. My patience was non-existent. I was short with the departing nurse and even shorter with the CNAs coming on shift. I traded in my optimistic thinking for negative thoughts and self-pity. I needed a time-out. I identified my toxic behavior and knew that it was wrong and completely unproductive. Identifying bad behavior is one thing but doing something to change it is a completely different animal. I could keep letting it get the better of me, or do what I'd learned in my Alcohol Support Groups. I decided to take that time out and pray and meditate. It always worked in the past and I decided to rely on it once again. I walked into the four-by-four med-room next to the nurse's desk and let the door close behind me. A CNA called me for something mundane and unimportant and I ignored her. I shut the light and said my arsenal of prayers. I had just said them on the train on the way here and even sitting by the pond again, but my spiritual gas tank was already depleted after hearing of another monster assignment. Due to the recent self-slavery that my mind was battling, I needed prayer badly. I said the Serenity Prayer, the Lord's Prayer, the Hail Mary, and two Alcohol Support Group prayers. I also asked God for strength and patience. I asked for a safe shift and the ability to work well with others. I asked for clarity and wisdom. I asked to live in God's light and carry His love.

I breathed deeply and visualized myself running through these resident's rooms, changing my PPE in and out, and in general, kicking COVID ass. If I was to survive this shift I would need to rid myself of the self-bondage my mind was imposing. I was worried about myself and the distress and hard work I would endure over the next eight hours. I concluded that I was being selfish and I needed to consider the residents and their feelings about being locked inside their rooms facing uncertain times.

After this impromptu prayer session, I felt embarrassed. How could I be so worried about myself when all the poor residents were prisoners in their rooms, terrified of this media-bloated and weaponized virus? My embarrassment turned to shame and disgust. I can't recall if I apologized to God in those moments, but He sure deserved one. I closed my eyes and took some more deep breaths and focused on the black behind my closed eyes.

I exploded out of the medroom with a new pep in my step. I focused on the future and getting through this shift safely and swiftly. I didn't focus on the shame I felt about my selfishness—it would get me nowhere. God had given me another chance at life and directed me to help His children and to do His will and I should be honored and humbled that He allowed me to do so. This was His plan for me. The power of prayer continued to keep me afloat on the viral lake of fire. The power of prayer was real for me, ever-present, and extremely important to my mental health. Without prayer, I would accomplish nothing, and if I did somehow manage to accomplish anything, I would have done so in complete mental anguish and agony.

It had been two days since Wally Lasiter had been sent down to quarantine with a fever of 102.1. I hadn't even thought of him or his well-being in the tornado of emotions I had felt when I'd come onto the unit. I prayed a quick one for him while I stood at my med-cart organizing. Wally was one of my favorite residents. During my first couple of weeks he'd given me a hard time, but then I realized he was just worried about his health, and I couldn't blame him for that. After a month or so he started to trust me completely. I learned his quirks and preferences and we became fast friends. He knew he could count on me to always be there for him and help him. He would sometimes wake up from a nap confused and delirious because of the psych meds he was on, and yell at me accidentally. I did my best to not take offense to these types of confrontations because I knew that it wasn't the resident talking but rather the caustic medications he was taking. Wally talked about baseball and would always update me on the delay of the 2020 season. There was nothing much to update me about but I listened and acted as if I was hearing the information for the first time. I knew Wally was strong. He had congestive heart failure, Parkinson's disease, and some other minor issues, but despite all of this he enjoyed his simple life and got plenty of exercise. For an elderly gentleman in a wheelchair in a nursing home, he was *in shape*. I was very worried about Wally's chances of surviving COVID because of his diagnoses making him the perfect candidate for the 'Rona Reaper, but I would not be surprised at all if he survived. Wally once told me he hadn't drank since 1982. I never asked him to elaborate, but I felt like we shared a bond. At one point I shared with him my sobriety date and he told me good job, and to keep it up. He also kept two bibles at his bedside and was a member of The Knights of Columbus so we had the spiritual thing in common too. I hoped I would see him again. I thought of Barbara Watkins and Agatha Monroe and was grateful no one else on my unit had been sent down.

On the refugee side, another person was sent to quarantine with a fever. Her name was Valerie Smith. She was seventy-five years old, weak and frail. Valerie was a corrections officer in the county jail. She could have been my corrections officer if I'd crashed my car a couple of miles down the road in the next county. I don't remember her diagnoses but I remembered both her hands were badly contracted. It made it difficult for her to do simple things the average person takes for granted. She had trouble using forks and spoons; depending on what she was eating she would use her fingers if it was easier. When her sister called we would bring her a portable phone, put it on speaker and rest it on her chest since she couldn't handle the phone without accidentally hitting every button. We talked about New York sports. She was a Knicks and Yankees fan. We trashed the Knicks and their management. We always said, "One day we'll be back!" Sometimes she would say something like, "Yeah, they'll be back, but I probably won't be." I would either pretend I didn't hear or say something like, "Oh, you stop that." The truth is I heard everything. Everything the residents said, everything the CNAs said- unless they were speaking in French, and every pin drop. If what I heard was something I didn't like or didn't know how to handle, I would pretend I was spacing out. If I heard something that needed addressing I would do so. I worried for Valerie and prayed for her. COVID was known for taking the old and sickly and she was another perfect candidate for the 'Rona Reaper.' All the residents were *perfect candidates.*

Subtract those two residents from my thirty-seven, and I was left with thirty-five. It was a sick thought, but I was slightly relieved I had fewer people to take care of. We were understaffed downstairs on quarantine because more and more residents were going to the quarantine unit. Since there were roughly twenty people down there at that time, they had to staff an extra nurse to help with the growing population. Each nurse would have around ten residents to take care of. They also had two CNAs to split up the work as well. It was still a tall order because of all the PPE and precautions. They wanted a lower resident-to-nurse ratio because the residents required serious observation due to their COVID prognosis. I wondered how Mike Donald would be doing now. And Evelyn. *Poor Evelyn.* With her luck, positive attitude, and strength she would make it through this.

I had started my med-pass with all these thoughts running through my head when I realized I really needed to focus. *Did I make any errors on Jan and Leanne?* If I did I couldn't go back now and take the medicine from their bellies. On to the next one. Adrian was angry as I woke him up for his medicine. He started accusing the staff of taking the soda next to his bed. I thought to myself that he was crazy, but then I considered it... if he'd been sleeping, anyone could have come in here and stolen soda—I recalled the millisecond when I'd contemplated it the night before. I'd heard of the residents' and even the staff's belongings going missing and blaming the other side, so I couldn't rule it out. Suddenly Adrian wasn't so crazy. It was a shame that the people working here could do such a thing. It wasn't my side of the street to clean anyway. Adrian took sips of soda in-between each couple of pills, much like the late-night routine we'd recently perfected. While giving him what seemed like two dozen pills I spontaneously started singing "This little light of mine." I tried to get his mind off the soda. He looked at me skeptically but kept taking his pills. I kept singing because it made me feel good.

As I was walking out, Jim Moss said to me, "David, you have a nice voice."

I was completely taken off guard... again. It was as if your beloved family dog just started talking one day. Jim had hemiplegia from a stroke and I assumed he was borderline non-verbal. He only ever answered questions with a yes or a no, so I was absolutely shocked and even more delighted when he paid me the unexpected compliment. "What!? Well, thank you, Jim! Did you like that song!?"

"Yes, I did," he said, and then closed his eyes. Maybe today was going to be a good day after all. I thought to myself about the recurring lessons I always had to keep relearning. Don't judge a book... don't assume... maybe some other ones in there. The point was that I'd never even tried to talk to Jim. I'd only asked him my standard three questions about pain and bowel movements. I'd only taken his vital signs and given him his crushed medicine in applesauce. I always told each resident what I was doing, even if they looked like they were completely unconscious or brain activity was completely absent. In my defense, even with my regular twenty-seven residents, I rarely had time for conversation. I still could have done more. My Haitian CNA, Iris, was outside the door, gowning up for the girls. I asked her, "Did you know he talks?!"

"Ooo?" She sounded like a Haitian owl.

"Jim, Iris! JIM! He was just talking to me!" I practically yelled at her.

"Yes Daa-vee'. Jim talk a lot. 'E lead singer in band." She was almost annoyed at my enthusiasm.

"Ah, I see!" I said as I started to move my cart. Iris wanted no part of this conversation, but this would explain why he enjoyed my little song! I started imagining us singing and tap dancing together for the whole facility with top hats, canes, and red and white barbershop shirts— and of course a face mask! Okay back to work!

With my newfound energy I bounced around as fast I could, pausing for gowning and de-gowning between each room. I started to sing my favorite band Dispatch from memory. I wouldn't give in to playing music through earbuds or even on my phone, but I'd be damned if I couldn't make my own! Some residents enjoyed it and some maybe thought I was mocking them and the dire situation they were in. If a customer wasn't happy, I switched to Old Blue Eyes. If they still weren't happy with Frank I would just stop. Tabatha was one of the residents who didn't enjoy my singing. I entered her room singing "Fly Me to the Moon," and stopped suddenly and looked at her as if her presence had surprised me. "Have you ever heard of this guy, Frank Sinatra?" I asked in jest, knowing it might make her mad. *Too easy!*

"Oh...My...God..." she said slowly as she rolled her eyes, "yes... I... heard... of... him!"

"Oh okay, yeah, I really like him." I was smiling ear to ear but she couldn't see it because of the mask. I got her good. Because of my comical and musical torture, I was especially nice on the way out. "Tabatha, do you need anything right now? I won't be back till 9 p.m." I switched to regular time because Wally was the only one who understood it.

"I... need... fresh... water..." she said, slower than grass growing, "I... haven't... had...water... in... three... days..."

"Three days?! Oh my! Okay, I'll be right back," I replied quickly as I de-gowned and ran out of the room. I knew she was going to ask for water and I knew I would have to fetch it for her since I made this mistake the day before with her. I figured I had to be nice to undo the fun I was poking at her. Since she was still in her wheelchair I could just crack the door open and leave the water on her roommate's dresser and she could come and get it. This saved me another wardrobe change and more plastic PPE wasted.

On my way back to her room, her neighbor Leslie Dawson was yelling about something. I dropped the water off and moved my cart quickly to Leslie and Barbara's room. Barbara wasn't there and maybe Leslie felt lonely. The door was shut and Leslie was at the edge of the bed ready to get up. I don't know where she was going. I don't think she knew either. Her mind was completely gone. If I had been down the hall she surely would have gotten up on her own, taken a few steps, and fallen. She loved to get up and walk on her own. She loved to fall. Her bed alarm wasn't engaged because I would have heard it go off. Poor nursing for her bed alarm to be turned off. More nursing fundamentals that were overlooked, which would prove costly if the resident fell. Usually, when the CNA would change a resident's diaper, they would turn the bed alarm off because otherwise when they rolled the resident to one side it would sound the alarm. Good nurses would come running. Bad nurses wouldn't come at all. I turned it on and it started beeping loudly. I couldn't convince Leslie to lay back in bed. She wanted to use the bathroom. I conceded and took it upon myself to toilet her. I raised the bed and helped her get out. I walked alongside her with my right arm under her left. She was so unsure on her feet that it scared me. I preemptively opened the bathroom door on my way in, knowing that toileting might be the reason she *needed* to get up. We side-shimmied through as she held onto the door handle and my arm. Then she grabbed the sink and took a few more steps. She turned and put one hand on the side grab rail and the other hand on the grab rail in front of her. She went to lower herself and I loudly told her to stop. Before she lowered herself I had to pull her pull-ups down below her knees. Her usual look of terror returned when she realized she was in a bathroom with a man… alone. She was known for making rape accusations and I hoped she wouldn't start this type of thing now. I left the door slightly ajar so I could see into it. I went out into the room and straightened up what I could. I stepped one foot into the hallway and grabbed my cart and turned it 180 degrees so that the drawers were facing the inside of the room. I could prepare her meds from inside the room so I didn't have to take off the newly donned PPE. I got everything she needed and slowly went to the bathroom door and looked in. She was wiping. I went back and flipped through the MAR to the next resident's medications and decided to get them ready. I sanitized my hands with the pump bottle on my cart's surface. It was only a couple medications for Lucie Greer. I separated the little plastic med-cups so I wouldn't confuse the two. I went back to look at Leslie through the crack.

Unfortunately, she caught me and screamed, "Why are you watching me on the toilet!? Are you a pervert?!"

I panicked and embarrassingly thought that someone would hear and think I was indeed a pervert. Rational thinking won over the contorted notions in my brain. *Everyone knows Leslie has full-blown dementia. They know she's a fall risk. They know she says absurd shit all the time. They know I'm making sure she's safe. Plus they were all busy with COVID. No one was around to hear anything anyway. What if she makes an accusation?* My previous life full of trouble continued to haunt my thinking. I shouted at her, "Leslie! I have to make sure you get back to your bed safely! I'm going to come in and help you back to bed, okay!?"

"FINE!" She yelled back.

Sometimes you had to be very stern with residents. You had to tell them what it was and what was going to happen and why. Some would respond well, others would just get even more agitated. Leslie responded well to strong, sometimes intense direction.

"I'm coming in to get you," I said through the door. I stepped in and helped lift her by the armpits. I told her to hold onto the commode which sat over the toilet, and the grab rail on the wall. I lifted her pull-up to her waist and told her to wash her hands. She refused to use soap and dried her hands poorly. *Why did I even bother?!* I walked her slowly back to the bed with my hands under her armpits. She kept trying to grab onto an arm that wasn't there. I walked behind her because I didn't want her urine-filled hands touching me—I forgot I was covered in plastic PPE! I told her I had her six and not to worry, and continued to encourage her. It was a long eight-foot walk. I sat her down on the side of the bed with her legs dangling and told her to relax and breathe. She rolled her eyes. I then told her I would lay her down. I lifted her legs to the bed with my left hand while pulling her right shoulder towards me so her whole body would be straight in the bed. No doubt, all this activity would tire her out. I slowly lowered her bed down with the remote, and as soon as it came to its lowest position, she closed her eyes. I had to toilet residents like her because having to go to the bathroom is one of the main reasons residents who can't walk, try to. Crisis averted. I de-gowned, sanitized my hands, and got out of there. DJ Khaled came to mind and I said loudly to anyone listening, "Anotha' one!" Leslie stayed asleep.

Lucie was easy. She took her meds easily. I had to retake her roommate Julie's blood pressure three times. I started sweating after repeating the process the first time. All in all, I was in there for close to fifteen minutes. I finally got her blood pressure. Due to the parameters, I had to hold the metoprolol because her blood pressure was too low. Since I quit drinking I would rarely sweat. It was one of the many gifts of sobriety, but under all the plastic PPE, not perspiring was impossible. Sweating for me was an autonomic response to stress or panic. When things didn't go my way on my schedule and especially in a high-stakes situation like this, sweating was inevitable and I hated it. It made me feel dirty.

I was over an hour behind, due to all the extracurricular activities. It was impossible to do what was asked of us. When no one was around to help residents, I had to meet whatever needs they had. The ice water, finding the remote, finding the phone, finding the glasses, taking their shoes off, putting their shoes on, ad infinitum. With all the doffing and donning; and sanitizing of the blood pressure cuffs, the thermometer probe, and the pulse oximeter, I constantly felt like I was drowning.

I moved as quickly as possible down the hall. I still had eight of my residents to do, plus another ten down the football field hallway. I got my phone out of the med-cart and texted my two sisters and mother. They were all nurses and our group text was called "Shift Report." (If we were talking about our house plants and flowers we would rename it "Garden Club"). I texted them about how overwhelmed I was and how unrealistic it was to do thirty-seven residents' medications twice and also take vital signs on each one of them… twice! All of this in an eight-hour shift.

My two sisters and mother were resting safely and comfortably at home so they got back to me right away. They responded with, "I'm sorry, that's terrible," and "Refuse the assignment." They told me to do my best, and as for the vital signs, they said to leave the spaces in the MAR blank if I couldn't get to them. They suggested I just get temperatures on everyone since that was the number one vital sign that would show COVID potential. They were all veteran nurses so I heeded their advice. They also told me that skipping certain supplements wouldn't kill anyone. I started skipping multivitamins and omega-3 fish oil capsules. I also started skipping other 'medications' like throat lozenges. I also paid no mind to certain eye drops and nasal sprays. I reasoned that if the resident didn't ask for them then they probably didn't need them. I also reasoned that my facility was in no position to start firing nurses for such petty offenses. Nurses were calling out and taking leave of absences when COVID hit so we were few and far between. I started skipping vital signs as well and leaving their designated spaces in the MAR blank. I felt bad but there was nothing I could do. The amount of work in eight hours they asked us to do was utterly unrealistic and obnoxious. I started circling medications that I couldn't find and didn't have the time to look for. I became the nurse that didn't care about the MAR and signatures. I figured if there was ever a time or excuse to skip signatures and medications, the time would be now. And the excuse was a pandemic. I would never have a better time or excuse. I tried not to worry about the legal documentation or the lack there of.

I kept it moving and got to Jordan Cliff. He was particularly upset. He liked to get out of bed every single day and if he didn't get to, he would make it known. He couldn't get out himself and required a mechanical lift to place him in the wheelchair. The CNAs were also understaffed and overwhelmed, so plenty of residents were missed and left in bed. He would yell obscenities you couldn't understand until he got to the F-bomb. That was the one word he would yell with absolute clarity. Because he was upset, he refused to take his 1700 medications and refused his vital signs. I sat and argued with him for a good two minutes. It seemed like forever, standing there in his doorway yelling back and forth about the importance of at least taking his temperature as sweat continued to permeate my scrub top and leave moisture on the inside of each plastic gown I put on over and over again. I needed a shower already. I was angry, sad, and exhausted. He finally let me take his temperature and it read 102.5. *FUCK ME! Here we go.* I took off all my PPE, stepped out, and started to call the supervisor—then stopped right away when I realized they would want a rectal temperature to confirm the accuracy of his temperature. I put a new gown back on and new gloves. I had to change the thermometer to the rectal type. This would be a fun time for me and Jordan. He didn't want to do anything, I wondered how this would go down, so I just talked firmly and loud, practically yelling, (he was one of the residents who would be further agitated when trying to tell him what to do) "Jordan! You have a temperature! We have to get a rectal reading to make sure its right! I need you to roll over, lets go!"

"I don't give a fuck!" He yelled back at me staring right in my eyes while doing so. He reached a new level of anger I'd never seen before, but I matched his intensity because of the importance of this reading.

"Come on man! Here we go!" I tried to disguise my yell as encouraging and optimistic as if this task would be effortless for both parties.

He had hemiplegia so he could only fight back with one arm, but even his one working arm was weak. I rolled him towards his bad side so could grab the rail with his good hand. Once I got him started in care, he was *somewhat* compliant. I pulled his brief down low enough to get the thermometer in there. I had to turn the BP Machine back on because it had timed out and gone to sleep. We waited together in the awkwardest of moments. His face was turned away from me but we could both feel the uncomfortable moment as if it was a tangible object we were both holding. He was an alpha male and I was a quick-witted singing nurse. He must have lost all of his dignity every time he got probed by a rectal thermometer. The BP machine finally turned on, I took the thermometer and gently stuck it in his rectum. He jumped a bit, then squirmed, and I yelled, "Stay still! We're almost done!" The machine beeped. I turned my head to see 103.4. Almost a full degree higher than his oral temperature. I would have to stop my med-pass, call the supervisor and book a room for a two-week COVID quarantine stay-cation.

Desiree was the supervisor. She had been a nurse for less than a year and apparently, was the best we had. She was an RN and was newly promoted to evening supervisor just days before. I spoke to her on the phone and could tell she was panicking. She probably had a thousand other things going on. My instructions were to keep him in the room with a mask, auscultate his lung sounds, and continue to monitor his oxygen levels. She told me she would come up as soon as possible to move the resident. She had to first confirm there was a special air mattress in an open room downstairs in 1B that Jordan required. By this time, the quarantine unit was quickly filling up. Apparently, most of the cases were coming from all over the second floor now. Someone was spreading the virus around, not knowing it. It was a waste of time to postulate who it might be. It was already in the building spreading like a wildfire.

I focused on what I could and continued my doomed 1700 med-pass. It was close to eight o'clock by now. I figured the only thing I could do at this point was to consolidate the 1700 and 2100 meds and give them all at once for my refugees down the football hallway. The remaining original two residents of mine would get the same modus operandi before I departed my hallway. I was walking back towards the hot corner and my nursing desk. It was a war zone. Ripped blue plastic gowns covered the floor. There were used gloves everywhere. Bags of dirty linen were piling up. It was absolutely disgusting and even more depressing. Housekeepers, CNAs, nurses, linen department—everyone was calling out or not even showing up. The remaining staff was forced to work overtime in this increasingly depressing facility. I went to the refugee residents and did the best I could. I was tired. My feet were on fire. My legs were throbbing. I was hungry. I hadn't eaten anything since getting to work.

Thinking about my empty stomach made me hungrier. I found a banana in the kitchenette and ate it as I walked down the hundred-yard hallway to get the other med-cart I had to share. Luckily it wasn't being used so I just had to find the nurse with the keys to it. She was nowhere to be found, and I didn't even know who it was so I couldn't call out her name. I walked down to the cafeteria/dining room to see if I could find the nurse and maybe some more food. The facility did provide meals for the staff. Sometimes they were good, sometimes they were barely edible. I found a mystery meat slab with mashed potatoes and green beans. I didn't even reheat it. I ate it standing up within sixty seconds.

I walked down to the massive but deserted central nursing station. I waited a minute, looking for my nurse, and then decided to walk slowly down the hundred-yard hallway waiting for anyone to surface. If I found a CNA they would be able to tell me the name of the nurse and I could start calling. Madeline, the CNA, popped out of a room and told me it was Cathy. I started yelling for Cathy immediately.

"She downstairs Papa, don't go yelling now!" the aide was surprised I was yelling. I'm not sure why she was surprised—everyone was in foul humor these days.

"Oh sorry okay, when is she coming back?" I asked, embarrassed but laughing. I should have asked the CNA where she was before yelling the nurse's name.

"She took Peter Richey down, 'e had a feeva," she told me as she started to walk down to pile more linen on the growing mountain of soiled items.

I thanked her and continued down the remaining fifty yards to the hot corner. I thought about the two more residents going downstairs—Jordan Cliff and Peter Richey—eventually, another quarantine unit would have to be opened.

I got to the hot corner which was also deserted and quiet and sat down and prayed. I prayed for more strength and patience. I prayed for the staff. I prayed especially long for the well-being of the residents. I mentioned Evelyn and Wally in my prayers too. I closed my eyes and focused on the black. I put my feet up on whatever I could and tried to rest for five good minutes. After less than that, I heard someone coming down the hallway, jingling keys.

"Oh, David?" Cathy called out like a game of hide-and-seek. She seemed in a good mood even with her gigantic assignment.

"YES!" I shouted out, fearing she wouldn't hear me, and she'd turn back around and leave. I popped up on my feet and hustled around the desk.

"CNA told me you were looking for me? You need the keys?" she asked excitedly, like she was dying to get rid of them.

"Yes, I still gotta do my whole half of 2BC. Are you done with yours?" I asked, half hoping she'd somehow done all my extra residents and was going to surprise me.

"Yes, I finished them. All yours!" We didn't count the narcotics. I trusted Cathy and she didn't look like a drug addict. She was older and Filipino. She'd probably never touched a drug in her life. This wasn't great reasoning because addiction affected everyone regardless of race, ethnicity, upbringing, or culture. In addition to all that, mistakes could still have been made either way, and Cathy and I would get in trouble for any narcotics that might be missing. Since I was being monitored by the Board of Nursing of New Jersey, I had to pay extra-special attention to handling and counting of the narcotics. I had no time to count them though, so I took the keys and started my med-pass on the remaining eleven residents. I wondered what type of Filipino magic Cathy possessed to get through thirty-eight residents in less than four hours. I wondered if she was coming back for the second med-pass at 21:00. I wondered if she skipped certain residents who didn't have any important medications. More speculation and wondering got me nowhere. I got to work.

I was halfway through when Desiree came to get Jordan Cliff. She asked me a dozen questions. I answered them as best I could. I told her the lungs were clear and his oxygen was 97%. I told her how the only sign of COVID Jordan had, was the fever. She double-checked my work and confirmed the oral temperature was still in the 102 range. I told her about the rectal temperature and how I had administered Tylenol immediately. She was impressed that I went that far and thanked me for it. I felt proud. I was a brand-new nurse but I was checking all the important boxes, asking important questions, and implementing important interventions to keep my residents safe. Since I'd gone to school six years earlier, I thought I would forget everything. I forgot a lot, but a lot of the important stuff was ingrained in my brain.

She took Jordan down and I wished him good luck. I didn't have much sympathy left that day. I found it difficult to genuinely care for someone who cursed me out on the regular, let alone during what my coworkers and I were going through. It was a cruel thought, but I remember thinking I didn't care if he lived or died, and I wouldn't waste any time or prayers on him.

The rest of the night was no better than the first five hours. Miraculously I got done with all my duties, except for the second set of vital signs. I did my treatments and got out of there. A CNA made me laugh on my way out. She was talking about the second floor being a ghost town. She said it in her Caribbean accent and I thought of New Orleans and Haiti and voodoo and it tickled me somehow. I was glad to be leaving the building while laughing.

I unlocked my bike and pedaled hard down the roads to the train station. Ghost roads, ghost trains, ghost buildings. Everything was sad. I saw a couple of cars. I prayed for the strength to keep this impossible pace up. I then remembered something I heard in Alcohol Support Groups, "God never gives you more than you can handle." I'm not sure I believed in this saying. You basically had to handle whatever came your way, so the saying was always true… it was almost a paradox. I compared the slight deception of this saying to what you'd tell someone who lost something. "It's always in the last place you look." These things made me chuckle in my head. I prayed for my family and that they stayed home and stayed safe. I prayed for all the residents and staff and all the essential personnel going to work each day. I included all the grocery store workers because they couldn't take any days off—people had to eat. I prayed for Jordan Cliff and asked for forgiveness for my lack of compassion for him and his situation.

Chapter 11

April 5th-April 15th

Without a dull and determined effort, there can be no great and glorious achievement- Xun Kuang

Over the next ten days, I worked seven shifts. Every shift was overloaded with residents. I always had over thirty-two residents. As more and more residents moved to quarantine, the deeper I went down the football hallway. By the end of this period, I had residents at the 2C central nursing desk, all the way down to the hot corner and down to the end of my forty-yard hall. By the end of this period, we sent down another fifteen residents from this floor of the building. Another dozen from the other side of the floor went down. Now the other half of the first floor was also quarantine. 1A— quarantine—two nurses, two CNAs. 1B—quarantine—two nurses, two CNAs. Each quarantine unit had approximately twenty-six residents. The second floor still had over sixty residents divided by two nurses and three or four CNAs. Many rooms were empty in between the occupied ones. Sometimes I would care for a resident and leave and have to travel three rooms—or approximately twenty yards—to the next room with a resident in it. We had lost two residents by this time and there were murmurs of another two not doing so well.

After the third day or so of working with thirty-two-plus residents, I found my groove. I got to know the refugee residents better and learned their dos and don'ts and their preferences. I learned what pills they absolutely refused. I learned time-saving steps and shortcuts. I thought that taking extra time to organize the refugee cart would save me ten times the amount of time in the future. I reordered all the medications that were missing and was able to really move during my 1700 and 2100 med-passes.

Whenever there was no regular on a cart, the cart became absolutely awful. It was disorganized; medications weren't reordered. Each shift was pure survival. Don't drown. Find the medication, pop it, administer it and throw the medication back in the cart. It was literally dirty as well as messy. The care for the residents without a regular nurse also suffered. Some agency nurses and part-time/per diem nurses could come in for a shift, give their medications and leave without doing much else for them.

By the time a problem was found it was hard to reverse it. When a wound was found it was very difficult to treat the resident and get them back to where they used to be. If the resident had a deficiency or a newly developing illness, sometimes it would be too late. The nurse just didn't have time to assess and inspect every resident thoroughly. They were too busy finding medications or gathering supplies they needed, or just dealing with utter bullshit a nurse shouldn't have to be responsible for. Units with regular nurses usually thrived. Residents got sick and injured, but if there was always the same set of eyes on them, you could spot problems faster and fix them easier and prevent further decline.

The benefit of having regulars on a floor is that the nurse knows the resident and the resident knows the nurse. This is called continuity and it is paramount in nursing. An added benefit is that the nurse can become emotionally attached or invested in their residents. I felt that happening with me. I cared deeply for several residents within the first two months of my nursing career. I could compare my feelings towards my grandfather with how I felt for some of the residents. This was a good thing because people got better care from someone who genuinely *cared* for them. Just as I got to know the ins and outs and preferences of the refugee residents I had picked up on my assignment, they would suddenly show signs of difficulty breathing or fever, and then they were off to the COVID quarantine floor.

On or around April 15th, Evelyn tested negative for the COVID and was welcomed back to her room. It had been terminally cleaned and a bunch of her belongings had been thrown out. Housekeeping and maybe other department heads including nursing must have ordered it. There were still many unknowns about how long the virus could survive on surfaces. I refused to believe that a virus could live on a surface for more than a couple of hours. The media kept repeating that it was possible for it to survive for three days without a living host. I thought that that was very unlikely, but if it were true, maybe this really was the apocalypse. Shame on the press either way—they never got the benefit of my doubt... ever.

A couple of other residents returned to their rooms up and down the hallway. I waited for my buddy Wally Lasiter to come back up but figured it might be a couple more days—maybe a week before he would test negative. That was another unknown about COVID. How long could the virus last in a human? How long would they be considered contagious? Since we didn't know, the resident would have to have a negative test before they were allowed to go back to their regular room.

On my days off I was doing push-ups and sit-ups, watching movies and TV series on Netflix with Candace, and hitting my online Alcohol Support Group meetings. I also had to do one Zoom meeting a week with my peer support group meeting through the Board Of Nursing. They hired a third-party company to move the meetings online and oversee the management of them. This transition was six months before COVID came around so when the Alcohol Support Group meetings took to Zoom, I was a pro and was able to help others who were having trouble. I remember being in a seventy-person meeting at the beginning of the Zoom era and setting my background to a picture of cacti in Arizona. People were confused, impressed, laughing, and generally entertained. I got dozens of messages complimenting my background and instructed those who wanted to do the same. The next week at least two dozen people had backgrounds. Golden Gate bridges, Eiffel Towers, and all other monumental photos and scenic landscapes were the backdrops for my sober friends. The alcoholic who needed meetings had no other option but Zoom. It wasn't the same as in-person meetings, but it was sure better than nothing.

Conversely, the Board of Nursing peer support groups were a nuisance and a time consumer. Mine was every Saturday at 3:00 p.m. Our meetings went well, but no one enjoyed them and no one got anything from them—it was mandatory that the impaired nurse attend. If you missed too many you would receive a one-year extension in the program. We paid roughly $1,200 a year to be able to attend our Board of Nursing Zoom meetings. We would recap what our week was like or if we were having any problems. We would talk about the increasing frequency of our drug testing. It was partly helpful for newcomers who needed guidance in navigating the nursing sobriety program. People who were three or four years into the program could give advice to the new nurse who was only two months into their five-year contract. We told them about the dos and don'ts of the program and told them to hang in there. Although the mandatory Board of Nursing meetings didn't help as much as the Alcohol Support Group meetings, the social support was still there and played an important part in encouraging the disheartened and struggling nurse who might still be trying to accept this new five-year detour in life. It was particularly hard for the nurse who was in the program and didn't truly have a problem with substance abuse. It was rare— but it did happen.

Despite the pandemic and the risk of infection, the BON started to increase the frequency of testing. I deduced that their reasoning was that our stress levels as nurses were higher because of the pandemic, and the chances of us 'picking up' a drug or drink would also rise with our stress. Adding a third drug test a month was the *real source* of stress for us. We had to go to urgent cares before or after our shifts, to give blood or urine. We had to sit in the waiting rooms for hours on our days off. Nurses were some of the few remaining professionals who worked non-stop through the pandemic, and most of us were constantly and consistently subjected to the virus. Despite our inevitable and ongoing exposure to the virus, the Board of Nursing of New Jersey paid no mind to the potential of spreading the infection. They wanted us to wait in crowded waiting rooms three and sometimes four times a month.

Despite my constant monitoring by the Board of Nursing, I didn't really have anything to complain about. I actually had something to celebrate. I received a $1,500 retention bonus from my facility. It was taxed, so I walked away with about $900 and change. I was elated to receive the monetary compensation. It still wasn't worth the ten-hour shifts covered in plastic and double-masked; I would rather be sitting at home collecting unemployment like the rest of the world. It was still a very nice and well-deserved surprise. The CNAs got money too—I'm not sure about the other supporting staff although I believe they also deserved something—at least the ones who showed up.

The whole country was sending food to hospitals for the staff working insane amounts of time. Our nursing home was forgotten during all that generosity. I wished someone was sending us food! My brother and sister-in-law sent my facility ten pizzas one night and everyone was so thankful. One housekeeper thanked me profusely and actually started to cry a little bit. I could tell everyone felt the pressure of the situation, not just the nurses and CNAs. The nursing homes were forgotten at the beginning but we were working just as hard as the big leaguers in hospitals.

Word was getting out about the increasing infection rates in all the nursing homes in the tristate area, and it was getting to the residents. They were becoming increasingly anxious and scared. Some residents considered it a death sentence and were reduced to an "It's only a matter of time" mentality. When I was faced with these residents I told them to knock it off and started to list all the residents who were surviving and coming back to their rooms. I told everyone about Evelyn. As soon as I did, the resident would cock their head, twist, and look at me with eyes wide with wonder and amazement. They wanted to hear more, but I didn't have time. I never had time. I could tell the good news made them feel better and made sure to keep spreading the good gossip, and never mentioned the death toll that was steadily growing.

By this time we'd lost three residents that I knew about. Two of them I had never cared for but had seen around. The third was Belle Montagne. She was eighty-nine years old and practically waiting to cross over each day. Her eyes were always closed, even when she was awake and wheeling slowly around the facility. Her eyes would finally rest eternally. I felt guilty and I felt sad but after I thought about it, I was grateful. I knew God would take her to His Kingdom in Heaven and she would suffer no more. This was a mercy death. She was somewhat active, but she had every disease in the book and was always dependent on staff for everything. She breathed heavily and was always uncomfortable. She always had an air of exhaustion about her. After feeling good about her passing I started to feel sad again that I didn't get to say goodbye. We didn't exactly hit it off, but her elderly face made me think of a cartoonish old person, which I got a kick out of. Not a malicious kick, but I just thought it was uncanny the way she resembled old people from cartoons I grew up on. We'd eventually developed a respect for each other and even had a laugh here and there. Since she had a ton of medications to be administered I always forgot something—the eye drops, the nasal spray—and she would always call me on it. I'd hoped one day I would be able to do everything for her flawlessly but after her death, I knew the chance of repairing my ego with a perfect med-pass for her was gone. Although I wanted her to see my improvement, the fact that I was unable to say goodbye hit me harder than I expected. This would be a common theme in the months to come.

The other two residents had been similar to Belle's general condition. One had been completely bed-bound and the other could barely sit in a wheelchair by himself—after a few minutes his head and body would slouch to the point where it made you uncomfortable even looking at him. If it wasn't for the pommel cushion betwixt his legs he would slide right down to the floor. I heard their names and could put a face to each one, but never had a real connection. I prayed for all three of their souls the night I found out they'd passed to the other side.

Early April saw the trains running more frequently, but they were operating for essential personnel only. No one was ever on the train during the lockdown and the subsequent weeks that followed, especially at 11 p.m. at night. The conductors never checked my tickets, for fear of exposure. I wished I'd known they weren't checking because I wouldn't have spent the $60 on the monthly pass. I continued to call it the ghost train and took videos and posted them on my Instagram. The little bit of ego that remained inside me needed everyone to know I was still working on the front lines whilst they sat idly in their dwelling collecting their free money. It was also a strange sight to see such an empty mode of public transportation and I wanted to share it. I should have taken a time-lapse of my dark empty bike rides too, but never got around to it—I had a bike mount phone holder but never used it. Hindsight was always 20/20, even if the year 2020 wasn't.

I was wheeling a refugee resident of mine to the quarantine unit and he just wasn't having it. He was practically kicking and screaming as I did. The fear controlled every bit of him and it was manifesting in childish but understandable behavior. He finally calmed down when we got to the elevators and there were a few more sets of eyes on him. I suppose he also realized that his tantrum wasn't going to stop him from going to the COVID unit. He almost expected me to stop in the hall and say, *Okay, so if you really don't want to go, I won't make you* and turn around to bring him back to his room.

During the elevator ride, I shared a story of my alcoholism. He had already known of my sobriety and could relate to it because his brother was in the same Alcohol Support Group fellowship I took part in. I told him how, though it might look like the end, it could be a new beginning. "I know it seems that hope is lost but you just have to be strong and take it one day at a time. When I got sober I was falling down a deep, dark hole waiting for a jagged rock bottom. My life was shattered and I was ready to lose everything. Instead of a jagged rock bottom, a trampoline waited for me and I bounced back and became the best version of myself. Do you see what I'm saying? One day at a time! It's not a death sentence! Breathe deep so you don't get pneumonia—please remember that. And bounce back, damnit!"

The elevator doors opened right on cue as I wheeled him towards the looming double doors. I felt foolish because he just kind of shrugged and murmured something after my death sentence pep talk—it did absolutely nothing for his spirits or the mounting fear as we approached the gates of hell. His neutral reaction to my hopeful and inspirational speech was entertaining to me, though. We sat at the double doors which were covered in red posters and black lettering: "DO NOT ENTER" "QUARANTINE UNIT" "STAFF MUST BE IN FULL PPE IN ORDER TO ENTER." I decided not to give up so I said a specific prayer for him out loud and asked God to keep him safe and strong. I could tell he appreciated that because when I was done his eyes were closed and his head was still bowed. Right on cue again, the CNA came to gather him and his wheelchair and wheeled him to his new home for the next two weeks. I shouted through the closing door, "Breath deep and bounce back!"

The CNA probably rolled her eyes but I didn't do it for her entertainment or approval. I hoped my optimism might linger in his mind and keep him afloat. If all he remembered was to breathe deeply, then the whole pep talk would be worth it. Pneumonia secondary to COVID did all the killing at our facility, not the actual COVID.

Work sucked and it seemed it would only get worse. The do-si-do of room changes continued and it was in favor of residents going to quarantine rather than coming out of it. Every day I continued to wonder whether or not it would get better. I kept telling myself that something had to give, and even if we lost a third of the population like what happened with the plague, the madness would have to end eventually. It was torture and it was unfair and I was in the middle of it. Poor me. Poor me. Pour me a drink. This type of thinking and added stress would surely lead to my next drink. I could only take it one long, exhausting, sad, stress-filled day at a time. Two more residents passed away in mid-April, bringing our new total of COVID deaths to five. I did my best with my immensely heavy daily assignment and found my groove. I tried not to focus on the ones dying but rather on the ones surviving and getting back to their life in the nursing home. I was still fatigued and waiting for the tide to change. It finally did. Hope and actual physical relief finally came...

Chapter 12

April 16th

God always puts me where I'm needed - Traveling Nurse

At last! We were saved! Travel nurses and CNAs came from all over the country to help us. Experienced veteran nurses and hardworking 'take no shit' CNAs came to our rescue. I felt like a survivor of Katrina in New Orleans or a shipwrecked passenger on that island finally seeing the coast guard after weeks of being stranded. Every new traveler I met that night I thanked profusely for coming to our aid. They were compensated *very* well but they came knowing the risk of exposure. The main reason most came was that they were doing the right thing for people who needed help. We had travelers from New York, Pennsylvania, Maryland, Virginia, North Carolina, South Carolina, Georgia, Louisiana, Florida, Texas, Arkansas, Mississippi, West Virginia, and Oklahoma. I'm sure I missed a couple of states but you get the idea. Fun southern accents filled our halls. The 2C monster desk would now be filled with nurses and CNAs from all walks of life. Before their arrival, we had mainly Haitian and Caribbean staff during the day and predominantly Filipino staff at night. Now our new and growing team were predominantly American-born.

Our new guests brought with them great work ethics and positive attitudes and renewed our spirits. People actually cared about us and recognized that we were in deep trouble. I was so happy I could cry. For the first time, it would have been tears of joy and not of despair and sadness. I'm guessing Governor Murphy approved emergency funding for all healthcare facilities to hire travelers—or maybe it was at a federal level—we didn't care. Our regular Nurses and CNAs were calling out for weeks at a time with the virus. Some employees left altogether to avoid contracting the virus and bringing it home to their children. There was no way we could have kept that pace up without terrible things continuing to happen and increasing in frequency.

Everyone rejoiced at their arrival. I was truly touched when many of them said that they heard the call from God and had to come help. *Use whatever gifts God gave you to be of service to others.* The first travel nurse I met was a thirty-something old man from Florida named Blake, who left his full-time job as a deputy in a sheriff's department in northern Florida to come help. He had been a nurse for a few years and then went into law enforcement. He hadn't practiced in five or six years, but his expired nursing license was reactivated due to the crisis in New Jersey. The tristate needed bodies and even some nurses were coming out of retirement to help. Somehow and once again, as one of the least experienced nurses in the facility, I got the job of training and orienting Blake back to his old profession and to our facility. *Who is putting me in charge of this shit? I wish they'd stop!* I let him do injections and G-tube medication administration in order to shake the rust off. I remember letting him watch me give one subcutaneous insulin injection and he stated that it all came back to him and he would be fine. With his extra hands and my guidance, we banged out my assignment's med-pass. I would prep the medications and he would take vital signs and administer them. We immediately had a sense of camaraderie and enjoyed each other's company. I told him that the alpha males had to stick together and keep everyone in line and he laughed out loud. Everyone was giddy as laughter and loud chatter started to fill the hallways. When entering a room with Blake, I would introduce him as my step-brother or long-lost friend from the army. We would tell the residents we were kidding, and they'd get a big kick out of it. The residents went from being confused about all the new personnel to entertained at our 'getting to know everyone' period with the travelers, and then back to their miserable selves. No one could blame them for their misery, but the first couple of days when the travelers arrived, provided a well-needed distraction from the subpar care the residents were receiving and the sad spirits that accompanied each employee into the residents' rooms.

That first night the travelers arrived, I had my first COVID departure.

It was the first resident on an assignment of mine that died. It would not be my last. The new total of COVID deaths was six. It wasn't a confirmed case and he never made it to quarantine. He didn't have a fever but had difficulty breathing. It seemed he was drawing shallow and slow breaths the moment I started my shift. The resident was an elderly man whose oxygen was desaturating. He was a DNR and bed-bound. He was another one who had every disease in the book and was already knocking on heaven's door.

As soon as I left the room I ran into another nurse stationed on the floor as a utility/desk nurse. I explained to her the situation and she said she would take care of it. She was from Oklahoma and was confident so I let her have at it. While she was walking away she said something about how God always put her where she was needed; I thought it was a beautiful thing to say at that moment and it couldn't have been truer. It could explain why I got my nursing license and job just in time for the first pandemic in a hundred years. She entered the room and sat with the man for ten minutes. She left the room, did some other work, and *returned* to sit with him and hold his hand. She kept that up for the next two hours. We kept him on oxygen but it didn't really help. Eventually, she told me that the man had passed away holding her hand. I walked into the room to check and make sure as if maybe she'd got it wrong. I felt like a fool walking out past her. She took no offense but almost looked like she was waiting for me to say, "Yup, you're right. He's dead." She told me she would call the family and the doctor, and wrap the body. I was so thankful I didn't have to deal with all that yet, I wasn't exactly ready. I would have had to do it alone if the travelers hadn't shown up. Maybe God didn't give us what we couldn't handle.

Since the travelers came we were fully staffed and then some. My resident count went from around thirty-seven to sixteen. The CNAs had eight to ten residents each, compared to the twenty a shift they were used to for the first three weeks of the COVID outbreak. Not only did we have dozens of extra bodies working alongside us, but they were also quality workers who had years—sometimes decades of experience. These were the nurses I would truly learn from. Not to take away from my regular coworkers, but at the end of the day, all the regular staff nurses did was administer oral and G-tube medications, and a few injections. I could hardly call it nursing. I joked with friends and family and told them I was a geriatric babysitter or even a geriatric drug dealer. My job was telling people not to walk on their own and arguing with them to take their medications.

That night I was stationed on 2A which turned into a quarantine unit that very evening. Three quarantine units now. The virus showed no signs of stopping as more and more cases were being reported. Practically all the cases that went to quarantine with a fever tested positive for COVID days later. I did hear of a resident who was unnecessarily quarantined with a fever and tested negative. He was brought back to his room once the negative test came back, only to test positive seven days later and go back to quarantine. Did he get the virus by being in the quarantine unit? Or did it just take an extra week to register on a COVID swab test? When residents moved around so much, their MAR records would get lost and their medications left behind. Since the medication was left in the COVID quarantine unit, we were not allowed to go and retrieve the medication. The pharmacy couldn't send more medication because the insurance wouldn't pay for it until a certain date. This was a mess and one of the minor problems we experienced in my facility during the pandemic. *If* we could get the nurse on the phone we would need her to locate the medicine and then coordinate when she could bring it down to the double doors to give it to the nurse who needed it. We weighed how important the certain medication was and whether it could be borrowed from someone else who was on the same medication on the same cart.

On 2A I met a nurse from Texas named Shawna. All I could see were her eyes and they were very pretty. For the first couple of days, I was very nervous around all the travelers. I thought I would be found out for the alcoholic, fake nurse I really was. I was always waiting for them to say, "What?! What did you just say? Did you even go to nursing school? Why would you do that?" I constantly thought I would be exposed. What was I doing here taking care of human beings? Fortunately for me and my ego, that conversation never came. Once I found out Shawna was from Texas I didn't ask her *if* she had any guns, I asked *how many* guns she had. She laughed and told me two. She asked me where things were and asked me about certain residents. I answered the best I could. We became friends during that shift and we helped each other out. She taught me nursing things that

I probably should have remembered from nursing school and other veteran tricks and tips that could only be acquired through experience and learning from other skilled nurses. She treated every resident like her grandmother. She genuinely cared for each one and let them know it. She would enter the room bubbling with enthusiasm and a warm southern accent, "Hi honey! My name's Shawna! I'm your nurse tonight! You feelin' okay, sweetie?" Most of the residents responded really well and enjoyed her company and the way she cared for them, especially the men—but then there were some residents that were never happy with anything. I was kind to all my residents but in many instances, I didn't really know or understand them. I certainly never shared a connection with most of them and I could be very short and to the point, especially during the weeks that preceded the relief we received. There was no kindness or love in my voice, I spoke somewhat monotonously and tried to let the resident know that I had no time to waste, but I was there to help. Shawna had a priceless southern charm that everyone was attracted to. I think a lot of the residents were confused about all the new southern accents coming into their rooms. Maybe they thought they'd been transferred to an Alabama facility overnight.

Shawna was the real deal; she knew every nursing skill in the book. Straight catheterizations, foley catheterizations, supra-pubic catheterization changes, G-tube placement, tracheostomy cleaning, and inner cannula changes. She could change ileostomy bags and securely place a CPAP or BiPAP machine on a resident's unwilling face. She was an IV insertion master. She eventually earned the nickname of sharpshooter because she could find any flat, non-existent vein and adeptly insert the IV needle and catheter. Since she also owned guns we joked at the fact that she probably was an actual sharpshooter when it came to firearms as well. Many of the newly acquired nurses excelled at all these skills. In these situations before the travelers' arrival, you would have to call each unit to find a nurse who was comfortable doing one of these procedures if you'd never done it before. Even if they were comfortable doing it, it didn't mean they were good at it or had the time to help. Now we had experienced nurses at every post willing to help and teach new nurses like me and to get their hands dirty. Shawna did it all and did it with a smile on her face. We talked here and there that night but rarely had free time. We were busy with our residents, our PPE, and our double sets of vital signs.

By this date the total number of presumed positive and confirmed positive cases was probably close to a third of our total resident population. The presumed positives were just waiting for COVID nasal swabs to confirm the diagnosis. Although our assignments went down by the count, it was still exhausting. If it wasn't double sets of vitals every four hours, it was the PPE constantly being put on and taken off every five minutes. If it wasn't the PPE it was a new fever or difficulty breathing that we would then have to fully assess and move to quarantine. If we weren't moving someone to quarantine, we were receiving someone coming out of it. If it wasn't the musical chairs, or in this case, beds, it was trying to make the residents happy. It was always something but at least we had help and the task suddenly wasn't as daunting as it had been for the first two weeks. I felt like a soldier whose platoon was cornered and about to be ambushed, when finally at the last minute, air support arrived to save the day. The evening news had stories of jumbo jets showing up with hundreds of nurses and CNAs reporting to the tristate to work the area's hospitals. The news anchors failed to mention how the nursing homes were also receiving some of these selfless nomadic heroes.

That night wasn't so bad. I had actual help from Shawna and CNAs who had no fear of COVID and came to work their butts off. I didn't have to ask a CNA once for anything. All the residents were clean and taken care of. Between the new support staff I had, the couple of days on COVID by myself, and the last two weeks of taking care of nearly forty residents a night, I felt a new confidence in myself. I didn't let it get the best of me and would never let it turn to cockiness because I was always one step away from making a blunder of things. Confidence was good in any industry, especially health care. If you walked into a room uncertain of something, a resident would pick up on it immediately and start to worry. They would ask, "How many times have you done this?" or "How long have you been a nurse?" and my personal favorite—"Do you know what you're doing?"

I was less uncertain about things. I did the best I could and adopted an attitude of: Keep the residents alive, check on them frequently and keep them as happy as possible—as happy as a prisoner could be. Life had gotten exponentially better in just one day. We had real relief and things were looking up, but so were the COVID infection rates.

Chapter 13
April 17th

Fear is the mindkiller - Frank Herbert

Just when I thought it couldn't get any better, we heard of all sorts of promotions and deals Corporate America was sending our way. Nurses could get a free meal from McDonald's daily. Free coffee from Dunkin' Donuts and Starbucks. The cop nurse, Blake, was going to McDonald's every day for his free meal. Marriott hotels were giving free rooms to "Health care heroes" for a month or two. Traveling nurses and CNAs began to occupy the vacant hotel chains offering free stays. Many of the travelers switched to Marriott for the free stays so they could save their entire lodging stipends.

Finally, local restaurants started to remember the nursing homes and I'm sure a great deal of this is owed to the media who repeatedly told the stories of the nursing homes and their grim outlooks. We got dinner from a Hibachi restaurant every night for at least three weeks. The food was always hot and always delicious. This generosity went a very long way for someone who was working tirelessly and feeling under appreciated. We also received meals from Lila's Diner which was on the interstate somewhere. I had heard of it before but had never been. Needless to say, their food was also delicious and immensely appreciated.

Apparently, everyone was receiving government money from the shutdown. Restaurants were no different. They were getting government aid to keep their doors open and their workers employed. Most restaurants had a facility that they were supporting and they would get those meals and hours subsidized by the government. I'm not sure exactly how it worked but we were certainly grateful. The Director of Nursing was the one handing out the dinners for several nights, and I was never exactly sure why. I assumed she had real work to do but chose to surrender her Nurse Practitionership and Director of Nursing title to become a cafeteria worker. She was never available for staff and sat in her office with the door shut for most of the day but suddenly took an interest in dishing out the free food.

All the vending machines had been empty for weeks now and no one was coming to replace the soda and snacks, but many of the residents wanted their soda and juices. I decided to go out on a limb and ask for donations from my friends and family on Instagram. I told them what was happening and how all the residents asked for soda but could get none. I put the post up at 9 p.m. or so the night before and woke up to $250 in my Venmo from all the Instagram viewers. In another couple of hours, I had raised a total of $450 for soda. It was an incredible response. I had my brother-in-law buy all the soda from Sam's Club the next day. I still had an extra $100 left over to spend on the residents. I would eventually buy a couple of high-end pillows and bed wedges for several residents. I was proud of myself and so happy that all my friends and family were such stand-up people. I had asked for two to three dollars from everyone and expected maybe a hundred dollars and was pleasantly shocked at the outcome. The residents would have soda well into the summer.

The next day I arrived on time and stopped at the check-in, in the lobby. I was energized from the donations I got and was practically riding the feeling like a surfboard. I went to the impromptu conference/locker room and got all my PPE. The wait to get checked in and dressed was much longer now that we had an extra two dozen people in our facility for each shift. I walked up the stairs and entered the monster 2C nursing desk area. It was especially full at this time because all the extra employees were changing shifts. Opening the door, I heard the yelling right away. It was Shawna the Texan nurse *screaming* at a six-foot CNA, "I don't care when your break was! You don't leave a person like that!"

"I already changed her today, I'm leaving now!" the CNA screamed back at her in front of an audience of about fifteen people.

"How dare you?! You should be ashamed of yourself! Is that how you would treat your mother?!" Shawna was screaming at the very top of her lungs. I was sure she could be heard fifty yards down each hall on either side of the nursing station. The CNA left through the stairwell and Shawna went to the nursing office, no doubt to report the injustice.

I was impressed and grateful that someone spoke up. I had seen similar instances with my CNAs, but I would rather change the resident myself than get into a confrontation like this. I was too new a nurse to be blowing up every time a CNA didn't do their job. This would win me no respect or love with the CNAs who had been there for twenty-plus years. Shawna continued to be the real deal. *I need a girl like that,* I thought to myself while forgetting about Candace at home. I thought about how bad-ass she was as I walked to my 2B non-quarantine unit.

By this time we only had eight residents in my original 2B unit, so I picked up another ten residents down the football hallway, which was fine. It was still much less than the census I'd been responsible for before COVID had happened, and much, much less than my assignment immediately prior to the traveler's arrival.

I arrived to find a Floridian nurse standing in Barbara Watkins's room. Apparently, Barbara beat COVID like so many others and was back in her regular room. Lana the nurse stood there with linens in her hands organizing and talking to Barbara. As soon as Lana saw me she asked me to come in. "David, can you come help me? We have to change Barbara; she's been lying in her own doo-doo for a little too long."

"Okay, one second," I said, as I put my bag down without sanitizing anything. *Ew.* "How did you know my name?" I asked, perplexed.

"Tanya told me that you were my relief today," she replied, laughing. "I'm Lana; nice to meet you!"

Two nurses changing Barbara—what a laugh. We got the job done in the same time it would have taken a CNA to do three residents. Bed baths and brief changes were the first skills we did in nursing school, but they were also the first ones we would forget once we started a real nursing job. The change itself was sloppy, uncoordinated, and comical but Barbara was clean and happy. Although it took much longer, we knew that she was as clean as clean could get. I asked Barbara if she felt better and she replied with a loud, smiling, "Aight!" She was more of a fan favorite now because of her recent bout with the Vid.

Walking out of the room, Lana said, "This CNA just left her sitting in all that. I told Shawna and she flipped out on her."

"Oh yeah, I walked into all that. They were screaming at each other at the 2C desk. The CNA deserved it though. What a piece of shit," I said, and then regretted the judgment I'd passed because I didn't know the full story. Although, I would have to side with my nursing comrade if I had to choose.

"Good. She deserved it. I was too scared to say anything to the CNA so I just let Shawna deal with it," she said, smiling but embarrassed.

I could tell she was smiling because her eyes were crinkled. She had acted—or failed to act—in this situation out of fear. I could relate to her apprehension and thought about how we as humans let fear decide things for ourselves and often outright run our lives. I would probably be guilty of the same offense in this same situation. I was still new to the game. Confrontations would come later after I had perfected my practice and my med-pass, and maybe once COVID was over. "That's okay, I'm sure she got reported to the supervisor and I'm sure she won't mess around with you or Shawna anymore," I tried reassuring her. She probably didn't need reassuring, *but what did I know!? And why would she listen to my dumb ass?* She stood before me as a whole nurse, RN, BSN, and with a load of experience. I had been a nurse for a little over two months. I laughed in my head about the thought of me ever giving direction to, or clarifying situations for experienced, hardened nurses.

The CNA was notorious for leaving her shifts early, and her residents unattended. They could be sitting in their own waste and she would be nowhere to be found. Apparently, she would take a break at two and never return. I began to consider how many times this happened each day all over the facility. I thought back to Shawna and the admiration I felt for her and her course of action. *That was some superhero shit! Or maybe it was just what anyone would and should do in that situation. Maybe one day I'll reach that level of kick-ass.*

I had a pep in my step that day. In addition to my low resident load, I kept thinking about the Shawna-CNA altercation and felt like the nurses got a win over the CNAs that day. I know that a lot of CNAs were watching the altercation. It wasn't about wins or losses or taking sides or nurses versus CNAs—after all, most of us were in the same union anyway—it was about being average when someone could do so much better. In my opinion, it was about people taking advantage of the elderly. Because Barbara was basically non-verbal, there was no squeak in her wheel. She couldn't yell or raise hell or demand to be changed. She didn't know any better, and if she did she couldn't express it; there was no urgency in changing her. Compare Barbara's status to a resident who was coherent and verbal, who could yell and scream and call the supervisor and get their demands met. No matter the cognitive or consciousness level, everyone should be cleaned immediately and treated with dignity. In my opinion, it just didn't happen like that. It was sad. Even I was guilty of it. During one night of thirty-seven residents and no help, I knew one was soiled and I knew it might be a while before someone got to change her, and I left her. A part of me died. Moving forward, I learned about priorities. The next time that happened, if a CNA couldn't get to her, I would change the brief myself and not worry if a couple of multi-vitamins and antacids were given fifteen minutes late.

Over a month into the pandemic lockdown the residents were still quarantined to their rooms, regardless of symptoms or fever or anything else. The nurses and CNAs were the only human contact they were experiencing. The doctors hadn't been in the facility in five weeks. The recreation department had stopped coming in around that time as well. The physical therapy folks were also sitting at home wishing they could work (this presented a whole other problem). Visitors had been banned since day one as well. Even the therapy greyhound that came to visit each Friday was no longer visiting his happy customers. My two-month jail sentence had been hell; I could only imagine how these people felt, confined to their rooms for five weeks and counting. In jail, I cooked for the officers' dining room and was allowed certain liberties. I called it culinary school because I spent ten-plus hours a day in the kitchen. We could do our own laundry and cut our own hair. We also had an hour of outside free time. We also didn't have actual cells since we were non-violent offenders. This lockdown had to be worse than I had it in jail.

Depending on the staff, their interaction with the residents could be short and meaningless or it could be everything to that resident that day. My fear of the virus was practically non-existent. I chose to believe God would keep me safe while I cared for his children—God and an n95 mask… and frequent hand washing… and constant PPE changes. I wasn't careless but I didn't care about Corona anymore. I was sure that *if* I did get infected my strong Greek/Irish genes would hammer it out over a day or two and I would be back to normal. I also thought maybe when I had strep throat I also maybe had COVID. I realized that I had wheezed a little bit for a couple of nights laying on my back. I also recalled that I still felt sick ten days into the course of the antibiotics. I compared it to the memories I had of having strep throat as a young boy and feeling better after the first two days of antibiotics. Maybe my strong genes had already kicked the COVID. Because of this newfound courage and my low resident count, I tried to stay a few extra minutes in each room entertaining the residents. Sometimes I would just let them ramble on about the sad state of the nation. Whatever they needed, I tried to provide it if I could. Some residents took advantage of my willing ears. One resident, Finn Weiss, had a knack for visiting memory lane—he had a lot of property there. He would tell me of times when he'd stabbed and slashed rival drug dealers. I told him I preferred the happier stories of his entrepreneurial spirit and how he would rent a van, drive to Maryland, fill it with crabs and drive it back to sell to Jersey restaurants. I would be standing in his doorway for a half-hour at a time listening to him ramble. All I could say was, "Wow!" And "Really?" Each shallow response I offered would earn me another story or explanation…

I started my 1700 med-pass with great gusto and speed. I did Leanne and Jan but failed to get their vitals. They'd come back to their room a couple of days earlier. I suspected because of their lack of human interaction, they were especially grouchy. Jan told me to "Fuck off" in a dozen different ways so I couldn't give her her meds. Leanne took the first spoonful of applesauce and Depakote and said, "That tastes…*TERRIBLE!*"

"I know, Leanne, but it gets better," I said, smiling under my double masks, knowing it was a lie. They were back to their usual selves. COVID survivors. Leanne took the rest of the bitter applesauce and I went my separate way. I did a simple jig while walking backward and Leanne laughed a little bit and said something about a tea party and marrying her. Jan Konkle kept screaming garbled obesities at me… or someone else.

Wally Lasiter was back and living life as best he could. Because all sports were suspended, he fell victim to Family Feud and Judge Judy. I tried to stretch his legs a bit because he was rarely getting out of bed. Upon seeing him for the first time since his COVID sentence I did my my best Will Farrell, knowing it would be lost on him. "Great Odin's Raven, Wally! Knights of Columbus, how I've missed you so!

Frank Duzen was enjoying his solitude. He took his few 1700 meds easily and went back to resting in his bed. I got to Jim and did his couple of meds in applesauce quickly. He was one of my best customers. He never complained. I decided to reward him with some singing. I chose one of my other favorite bands, "The Doobie Brothers," and their well-known "Black Water"…

Well, I built me a raft and she's ready for floatin'
Ol' Mississippi, she's callin' my name
Catfish are jumpin', that paddle wheel thumpin'
Black water keeps rollin' on past just the same

After the first verse, Jim chimed in with a deep smooth voice!

"Whoa black water, keep on rolling,
Mississippi moon won't you keep shining.

I was shocked and thrilled! Someone I could sing with! There was as much joy on his face as I'd ever seen. We kept singing for another minute or so. I saw Wally looking on in amusement, clearly enjoying the duet. We skipped to the end and sang about funky dixie land and pretty mamas holding us by the hand. Our voices got deeper as we sang in unison. It was one of the coolest experiences in my young nursing career. My mind went back to us in barbershop quartet red and white suits singing with canes and top hats. My mind also recalled what Iris had said about him being a lead singer in a band.

"Jim, you used to sing in a band?!" I asked.

"Yes. Lead singer," he said while making eye contact. I got a feeling he started to remember me more and more and with that came trust.

"Wow, that's great! What kind of music?!" I asked inquisitively. I wasn't sure if the questions were too much, but he kept answering them.

"Everything, David. We played everything," he looked up at the ceiling and closed his eyes.

I took the hint and said goodbye, telling him, "Okay, we'll sing some more later."

Tabatha Patterson was always in a foul mood and today was no different—as soon as I walked in she started yelling at me as if I was the one who'd imposed the isolation sanctions, "You're! ...treating!...us!. like animals!"

"I know; I'm very sorry Tabatha, believe me, I am," I said, knowing that debating the justifications about this isolation would do nothing but waste my time and energy. I could only validate her feelings and let her know she was heard. "It will be over soon; hang in there."

"It's!... not!... right!" she yelled some more.

"I know, Tabatha, I know." I gave her the meds and she looked at me with shock and offense.

"I'm!...not!... taking those!" she screamed at me louder and faster.

"Tabatha. You need these. I understand your frustration and I'm very sorry but I promise you'll make matters worse if you stop taking your medicine," I retorted quickly. It was a suave and informative reply. I impressed myself, but I started to sweat more than usual.

She rolled her eyes and huffed and puffed, but took the medicine begrudgingly. She didn't say thank you, which was unlike her, but I didn't care. I truly felt sorry for her. I thanked her and left. Whenever I thanked residents for taking their medication I always laughed in my head. They weren't doing it for me. They were taking their medication because their bodies and minds needed it. That average nurse would walk out at the first sign or thought of a refusal, to save time. The good nurse would take a minute or two to try and convince the resident to take them. Usually, I could outsmart or "trick" the elderly into taking their medicine. Morally, some might object, but people in healthcare would side with getting the meds down the throats of the residents any way they could... aside from using physical force.

Tabatha's roommate Ruby was not having any meds whatsoever. She would kick and scream and bite if you came close to her with medicine. I would wait till she started humming Silent Night later on. Maybe that would signal that she would be in a better mood.

Next up were Leslie and Barbara, my daily confidence was growing and growing with each resident and room I completed. I stood at the door putting on new PPE and through the crack, I could see Leslie at the ready to make a daring walk to the bathroom. I hurried and tied the plastic robe around my back and put some gloves on simultaneously yelling, "Leslie! Don't you get up!" She was shocked and surprised and looked towards the door for a second, and then finally located where the voice was coming from. She started crying and said something about wanting her mommy. I felt terrible and raced in there and asked her what was wrong. "Where are you trying to go, Leslie?" I asked sweetly.

"To the bathroom. Is that all right with you?!" She yelled back through gushing tears running down her face, frustrated, agitated, and confused.

"Yes, Leslie that's all right with me. I'll help you, okay?!" I tried to be supportive, sweat dripping everywhere.

"Who are you, and what are you doing here?" Her annoyance increased. A look of terror spread over her face.

"I'm David, and I'm your nurse," I said, putting my hands under her armpits and my right leg between her legs. "You do your best and I'll do the rest, okay?! 1-2-3!" I did most of the walking. I carefully walked 180 degrees to get behind her and positioned my hands back under her armpits once more. She walked very slowly, unsure. Any minute she could go down, so I bent my knees and straightened my back, ready to catch all her weight. We took six long, slow, suspect steps toward the bathroom.

I stepped to her side holding her right arm, quickly opened the bathroom door, and guided the same hand to the door knob. I ran back to her left side to support her, my left hand on her left arm, my right hand on her back and flank. She stepped into the bathroom. I guided her left arm to the grab rail and had her turn 180 degrees so her back was at the commode above the toilet. I put her right hand on the other grab rail to the right of the toilet. I had her hold the commode as I pulled down her pull-ups. I could tell she was uncomfortable with my presence but she didn't object. Leslie responded well to my stern direction most of the time, but I didn't need much this time. I lowered her down on the commode and left her on the toilet. No matter how many times Leslie and I did the bathroom ballroom dance, it was a new experience for her *every time*. I was a stranger to her *every time*. I started Barbara's vitals while I waited for Leslie to finish. I checked on her through the crack in the bathroom doorway and door. After a couple of times, she saw me and looked back through the crack. We had a brief staring contest through the crack in the door and eventually she asked, "Why are you watching me, you creep?!"

I held in laughter and replied, "Safety, Leslie. Safety!"

She didn't believe me, responding with a skeptical, "Yeah, my ass, you creep!"

Oh boy, here comes the accusations. "Just let me know when you're done!" I forgot I had tons of help so I checked out in the hall to see if CNAs were available. I didn't see anyone so I yelled half-assed, "CNA around?" I didn't want to yell too much in case someone would think it was an emergency. *Jokes on me, even if it was an emergency, no one would come!* Okay, that was negative unproductive thinking with some self-pity on top, so I stopped it. I checked her and she was finishing up.

She tried to get up on her own so I rushed in, scaring her half to death. "Hey, what's the big idea!?" she questioned me, yelling and maintaining fierce eye contact with me while the terror returned to her face.

"Safety, Leslie," I said monotonously while helping her up. I pulled up her brief and didn't check if she'd wiped adequately. We skipped the sink and the washing the hands part altogether. I walked her slowly back to her bed, ready for a mayday. She got safely in bed, took her meds, and took a nap. Same song and dance for me, brand new for her, never remembering any of it.

I finished her roommate Barbara, took off my gown in the room, trashed it, and left. DJ Khaled was back, and I shouted "Anotha' One!" while entering the hallway. One of the Mississippi CNAs saw and heard me and laughed, "Okay, Khaled!" We giggled and went about our way.

The rest of the night was okay, I had to send Corey Chapman to quarantine and he wasn't the least bit happy about it. I would say he kicked and screamed, but he was too obese to move his legs; he certainly screamed the whole trip through the hallways. He always threatened to call the assistant director of nursing. He remembered her name and even had her cell phone number. I tried to calm him, but it was no use. He wound up sharing a room with a gentleman he knew from the Friendship Club that served decaf coffee and donuts every Friday. I told him it wouldn't be that bad and we'd see him in a couple of weeks. I told him to think of it as a vacation. At one point he stopped his screaming and pondered this idea. His instinct got the better of him and he continued to threaten to call my supervisors and assistant director of nursing. I felt terrible for him, but half of me wanted to say, "You can call the ADON, she was the one who ordered this move!" I could tell his outrage was derived directly from the fear of the unknown. I continued to try to console him. He had the mind of a thirteen-year-old because of his severe mental disability. I listed all the people who had survived COVID and come back, and I told him of Evelyn—his vice president of the Friendship Club. He told me he didn't care and it wasn't right. I agreed with him but told him I couldn't do anything about it. I was just following orders. Corey was able to walk a step or two with support. He transferred from his bed to his wheelchair by standing for a couple of seconds, turning, and sitting with the help of a CNA. Corey would return to our unit unscathed from the COVID, but he would never return to his feet again.

After the exile of Corey, I went on to the next room, Luna Wolfe. I wondered if she had changed her name legally or if her parents were hippies. Whatever the case, it was a pretty cool name. I translated it to Moon Wolf. I remember I'd had her during one of my orientation days months before. She was completely miserable and morbidly obese. Up until that point in her life, she'd been living independently in her own apartment. She had multiple sclerosis and she'd had a bad flare-up that had rendered her legs completely useless. She had to call 911 and have the EMTs help her off the bathroom floor and to the ER. Since the hospital admission, she'd come to us for rehab but was in no shape to return to independent life. That first day I met her I'd seen bacon dog treats next to her bed and concluded she was eating the dog treats in-between meals for a snack. I'd been immediately disgusted. I never brought it up, it wasn't really my business—kind of.

Now she was a regular on my floor. I wasn't too thrilled at the prospect of another sickly resident. I got to know her and her medications a little more each day. She was actually very grateful for the care I gave her and always said thank you. I could tell her frustration was weighing her down completely. She always said how she shouldn't be in a nursing home at the age of fifty-nine. She constantly talked about other options and getting out of there. Her roommate was a woman named Elle Gustafson. Elle was funny and the two became fast friends. They talked about music and boys. They talked about staff and which ones they liked and didn't like.

Despite her attitude of gratitude, Luna was always saturated with her own grief and sorrow. I felt like I could do nothing for someone in such distress and emotional pain—even if I did have a cure or solution. I had no time to implement such measures. Her blood sugar was consistently in the 200s but she stated that she never ate. This angered and frustrated her further. I gave her her insulin and medicine. I asked if there was anything I could do while I was there. She said there was nothing and thanked me. Her gratitude definitely won points with me, since most residents rarely knew enough to thank us, or how much it could elevate a nurse's mood.

I wheeled my cart the length of the hall back to the desk. I wondered what I could do for Luna to cheer her up. No ideas came to mind but I felt a need to help. I'm not sure if it was how devastated she was about her situation, or maybe her young age. Normally someone drowning in their own self-pity, I would deem helpless and I would put forth minimal effort, but I decided not to give up on her. My only plan for her was to be extra nice and attentive when possible.

I got back to the frigid hot corner. It was empty except for a couple of CNAs sitting at my desk. CNA Mel was from Georgia. He was in his early twenties and acted like it. He made silly jokes, but his energy level was through the roof. He raced up and down the halls changing people and keeping everyone as happy as possible. Eventually, I would find him painting the female resident's nails and doing their hair. For the men, he gave haircuts in his extra time, even going as far as shaving silly mustaches on some of them. After doing double the work of the rest of the regular CNAs and all his recreational grooming, he still found time to sit and play on his phone for an hour or two. I was happy he had the time to sit and rest. I was grateful for someone who could match my intensity and energy and even exceeded it most times. I literally never once asked him to change a brief. They were always done before it ever became an issue. The residents raved about him. It wasn't all rainbows and unicorns though. The other CNA was Chanel, a young girl from South Carolina with an attitude and ego bigger than her home state. Every time I asked for something I got a roll of the eyes and an explanation as to why she didn't have to do it. I didn't work with her much, thankfully, but when I did I always dreaded the interactions. For the most part, Mel was stationed on my floor and we thrived. Despite all the help we got from the traveling nurses and CNAs, of course there came plenty of drama with all the clashing of personalities.

Chapter 14

April 18ᵗʰ

In addition to the two previous things a nurse needs to be good at, there is one more we need mention. That is public speaking! The nurse has to talk to the doctors, the resident, the family members confidently and swiftly... Presenting their case and getting what they need.

Just three days into the relief wave of traveling health care professionals, shit started to hit the fan. I could say 'literally,' but I'll choose not to, in good taste. The regular CNAs started accusing the travelers of not changing the residents' briefs. I could have laughed out loud when I first heard this. The travelers did double and sometimes triple the work in half the time, and they deserved to sit on their asses whenever they felt like it. The travelers, on average were probably twenty to thirty years younger than my regular CNAs. Most of the regular CNAs could trade their linen cart for a bed in our facility at any moment. They walked slow and worked even slower. In my opinion some of them weren't fit to work at all. One in particular needed a rolling bedside table to lean on while she walked; she suffered from kyphosis which is a concave curvature of the spine. She couldn't stand straight up any more and remained in a perpetual bow. I assumed the regular CNAs saw many of the travelers sitting and were confused as to how they could do all their work while seated. They didn't understand or see how fast the travelers worked, but figured they had to tell someone about it! This whole accusation parade went as far as having the assistant director of nursing come in unannounced on a Saturday night at 2200, to inspect residents' briefs. I'm not sure what the ADON found but I don't recall any travelers getting in trouble because of laziness or unchanged briefs. One resident was actually so used to being changed just once a shift that she was confused when a traveling CNA came to change her at 1600. She tried to refuse the early brief change because she thought that it would be the only change she would get for the eight-hour shift. She wanted to sit in her own waste for a couple hours more, letting it accumulate before getting cleaned, and that was what she was used to. Mel cleared up the situation and told her he would change her whenever she needed it, no matter how many times she went. The regular and traveler CNAs constantly and consistently butted heads. I told a couple of our CNAs, "You better enjoy it while it lasts and be grateful they're here! Once they're gone you'll go back to having fifteen residents a shift." They chose to ignore my unsolicited advice or maybe just didn't understand it. I'm not sure some of them understood that the travelers' presence was only temporary. I didn't try to clarify the situation for them.

The good times only ever lasted for so long. There was the inevitable COVID fever, quarantine or death. I heard of another two residents that had passed. Our new total was eight. I'd known some of them, and others, I had never even heard of.

The ones I did know were more of the same story. Residents with multiple heavy-hitting diagnoses. They were bed-bound with dementia. If they didn't have crippling dementia they had severe brain damage from stroke. They could hardly feed themselves. They were waiting to cross over either way. In these cases COVID was the angel of death. COVID took its victims quickly at the end. The signs and symptoms set in quickly, but were manageable for the first couple of days or so. Five to ten days after the onset of their symptoms came the toughest time for the them. Their breathing became more labored and they required more and more oxygen. Most residents who survived, got through this stage with ease and required no oxygen. The residents whose fate was already decided never made it through this stage. They often died alone and if they had family they might be able to talk to them on the phone once or twice before departing this material earth.

I was blessed to not have been back on COVID for a couple of days. They wanted RNs working on the COVID floors, instead of the LPNs. That was fine with me and for that period of time I was grateful I didn't have my RN. I wasn't scared of the virus but the workload and severity of the COVID units were immense. On top of the labor you also were emotionally and mentally exhausted. Worrying about the death of a human being and how they would say goodbye to their family was the hardest part for the nurse.

I heard staff talking about the lockdown and the quarantine. Everyone was upset that the two-week shutdown was still in effect. Everyone projected dates of when the country would fully reopen, or at least the tristate. COVID was running rampant through the country. A list of "hot states" was posted at the lobby check-in stations. If we visited these states we were supposed to self-quarantine for two weeks. I'm sure some would want the time off, while others wouldn't mention recent travels because they needed work. A lot of my coworkers were the only ones working in their family and unemployment hadn't really kicked in yet for their spouses or family members.

I thought about my family and how much I missed them. Since I was on the "front lines" and working in a facility with dozens of positive cases I couldn't see anyone, including my little nieces and nephews (but the Board Of New Jersey still wanted me in packed urgent cares, risking the spread of infection three times a month). I remembered the last time we were together was a couple weeks before the shutdowns in February. We were celebrating my sister's birthday, my nephews birthday and my birthday at an Italian restaurant on the interstate. It was a grand ol' time and I waited for the day we would all get back together again. I decided my coworker's projection of June first being reopening day was accurate and believed it, if just for a moment.

I counted the narcotics with the nurse from Florida. Lana was a good nurse and worked hard. We made jokes about certain residents and laughed at funny situations. She gave me a report of what was going on. There were still no MDs coming into the facility so new orders were few and far between. We also didn't have to worry about family visits. If you were on a COVID unit you might spend half your night talking to family members calling to check on their family each day. Some relatives called multiple times a day and even requested vital signs. You could talk to one relative and then have to give two separate relatives the same report later on. After a while if you sensed the pattern, you would have to tell the family that there could be only one person calling for updates because the nurses were just too busy to fill in Aunt Mary, cousin Joe and Uncle Ron during their shift.

Lana and I stood at the desk and continued to talk about our situation. We remarked how non-compliant the residents were becoming. Some residents started leaving their room more frequently and could make it halfway down the football hallway before a staff member saw them and yelled at them to get back to their room. Jared Bartell was one of these residents who did whatever he wanted whenever he wanted. He did comply with the mask wearing at least. If the residents weren't openly stubborn and defiant, they just didn't know any better. Frank Dusen probably didn't even know what a pandemic was or that we were in the middle of one. Lana and I sat and watched as Frank wheeled down the football hallway. He had slipped by the staff and was wheeling slowly past our desk. He had a mason jar of brown coffee and a fancy plastic box of sushi.

"Frank, what are you doing out of your room?" she practically yelled.

Frank stopped and looked in our general direction through his half-inch-thick glasses, "What?"

"You can't be out of your room, Frank!" she yelled back, looking at me, smiling through her face masks.

"Oh okay. I didn't know that," he said as he started to hustle in his wheelchair back to his room.

I thought maybe he was pulling a Keyser Söze, playing dumb like Kevin Spacey's character from "The Usual Suspects."

Lana laughed hysterically and sat down. I chuckled a little but didn't know why she thought pandemic non-compliance was so comical. I asked her what was so funny.

"He went to the refrigerator and took my coffee and sushi. That was my lunch!" she filled me in as she continued to laugh while rolling her eyes.

"What?! That was yours?!" I shouted as I sprang to my feet and moved towards his room. "I'll go get it, don't worry!"

"No, don't worry about it, let him have it. I don't want it anymore."

She kept laughing and asked if I could get the mason jar once he was done with the coffee. I told her I would try and we laughed some more. Frank looked like a rugged and tough fisherman, not a sushi and mason jar coffee kind of guy. We continued to laugh as she left.

Lana liked to get close to me and sometimes even touch me. She liked to flirt with me and I tried to give her no reason to continue it. We both had significant others at home; maybe she was just trying to pass the time and have some fun.

I started my med-pass with the scream queens. Each of them took their meds with ease. I guessed that Lana had been able to give both of them their morning meds. *Bravo, Lana!* The scream queens taking their meds in the morning generally made them a little more compliant throughout the day. They would also be a little less vocal and everyone appreciated that. Leanne told me how *terrible* the medicine in the apple sauce tasted, and I lied to her face saying it would get better, though I knew it never would.

I was in a certain kind of funk thinking about my family and wondering when I would see them again. I got to Wally, Frank and Jim's room and suddenly remembered how Jim and I sang the Doobie Brothers the last time. I thought of a classic rock song he was sure to know. I hobnobbed and dished out Wally and Frank's medication and then got to Jim. I was taking his vital signs when it hit me, "Black Dog," by Led Zeppelin would be the perfect selection. I loved singing this song and knew he would too. I sang as loud as I could, *"Hey hey mama, said the way you move..."*

Then Jim joined in and we sang together, *"GONNA MAKE YOU SWEAT, GONNA MAKE YOU GROOVE!"* Then we both made the guitar sounds best we could until the next verse, *"Ah-ha child way you shake that thing, gonna make you burn, gonna make you sting..."*

We did some more guitar sounds and then I had to take the lead for time-saving purposes. I skipped to the part where they say "Ah...ahh. Ah. Ahh," and I said, "Okay, I got to go buddy, we'll sing again later."

I thought he would be disappointed or sad but his expression stayed the same and he said, "Okay Dave. I like singing with you," as I shut the door. At least I was able to provide some type of joy during this pandemic of doom and despair, if not for Jim, then for myself!

I got to Tabatha and let her complain and shut her up with my combination of "Uh huh's, "I know's and "I'm sorry's. I tended to her roommate Ruby who was in a very hostile mood. She clenched her teeth when I tried to give her a spoonful of medicine. I thought of Mary Poppins and decided to sing her the spoonful of sugar song and what I remembered from it. This didn't tickle any fancy inside of her. Maybe she knew the song in German—I wasn't sure. I tried the medicine again and she angrily growled at me while still clenching her teeth. She then shouted *"NEIN NEIN NEIN!"* I knew this was German for *No!* and suddenly I was on the scene somewhere in Germany during WWII. I had one last hope. I would have to start "Silent Night" in soprano and see if it eased the tension. She had a seizure medication that she should probably take. Missing this dose would only make my life worse, or the next nurse's…

I took a deep breath and belted out my best falsetto singing a wordless silent night, "ahhhhh ah ahhhhh ahhh…"

She perked up and looked in my direction, "Ya, ya, zis is beautiful!" She joined me, and we hummed the second part together. Tabatha looked on in wonder and confusion, but the music we were making was actually quite beautiful and we sang in perfect unison. Tabatha enjoyed it. We sang on for a couple more seconds and then I rubbed Ruby's arm and said, "Okay, I need you to take this medicine for me," doubting my efforts.

To my surprise, she stopped singing and said, "Okay, yah yah," and took a spoonful of her medicine. Her face twisted and contorted at the taste of the anti-seizure medication and killed whatever moment we'd just had. She started spitting it out everywhere. I reacted quickly but then stopped. I was covered in plastic so I let her have at it. I can never get a win with Ruby. I tried my best. I suppose I could have tried again, but the VIMPAT is a counted narcotic and it might look like I took one myself or gave Ruby one too many. Regardless, Ruby wouldn't get her seizure meds that night. I hoped maybe she'd swallowed enough of the medicine for it to be effective. I would have to follow up with Tanya and see if there was a trick I was missing with Ruby.

I did Leslie and Barbara quite easily. Generally Barbara was pleasant and compliant and generally Leslie was nasty and required some finesse in taking her meds. Barbara always made me laugh; no matter what I said or asked her, she always responded with her ever-enthusiastic and high-pitched, "AIGHT!"

I got to Julie Walton and the recent stress melted away from me. She was non-verbal except for a rare, "Oh yeaaah." She wore a smile every time she saw me and it always made me very happy. If a smile could talk, hers would say, "Oh David, I know what you did," and she kept smiling even more as if my secrets amused her to the point of joyful insanity. I gave her her eye drops and wiped away all the goop from her eyes. It still gave me such satisfaction. I stood back and admired my work. Her eyes looked clean and refreshed now. At least I made a difference for one starfish, and the shift was still young.

I continued on down the hall until I got to the corner quadruple rooms where Luna lived and where Corey would live once he returned from COVID… if he returned from COVID. I was physically and emotionally exhausted. I was dripping in sweat. My scrub top was completely saturated front to back as it was every day. My boxers were also saturated, and I wondered if my swamp ass went through to my scrubs. People probably thought I shat myself. At least I was in the right place; after all, code browns were the norm at the facility.

I wondered what I would say to Luna to cheer her up. I asked God for clarity and wisdom. Luna's mood was about the same it had been for the last couple of days. She was still sad and still treading water in her own pool of self-pity. Self-pity was something I'd always been guilty of as a drunk alcoholic, but in my newfound sobriety it was one of the things that angered me the most. Since I'd been guilty of it, I could identify it so easily when I saw it in others, but I tried not to judge. I knew I had to help Luna but I didn't know why or what was calling me to do so. I anticipated her sour affect and glum mood so I had already accepted the challenge and was ready to deal with it. Mental preparation was always key. I gave her her meds easily. I checked her sugar—it was in the upper 200s— and I administered the insulin. She never caused problems when taking medicine, but her overall sense of depression depressed *me!* I asked her what I could do for her but she gave me no requests. It hit me on the way out, as I thought of her neighbor who was a double amputee from the thighs down. "Luna, I know it sucks, but at this point it can only get better!" I said quietly but optimistically. "It could always be worse, I promise you. You could be sitting here with no arms or legs. I know it's a weird thought but things could be a lot worse, okay?" I didn't know if using someone else's trauma to elevate someone else's mood or mindset was morally acceptable or even effective. I felt guilty about the amputee thing, not really knowing where I was going with all of it, but I continued, "Look at my bracelet— one day at time, that's all we can do. Let's get through today and see what happens tomorrow. If you need anything you let me know, okay?" I was out of breath and had no idea what I'd just said, but figured there had to be something of substance in that little tirade of motivational babble. I waited in absolute anxiety for her response and finally it came, "I know you're right, I just have to suck it up."

While leaving I said, "That's a great attitude; keep it up. I'll see you in a little bit."

I left before she could respond. I was out of ammo and out of ideas. Trying to pep-talk an older person with decades more life experience was very difficult and extremely uncomfortable. I compared it to the way I conducted myself around experienced RNs—I didn't want to say anything stupid or painfully obvious—but that was my ego being scared of how I would be perceived by my peers. I thought for sure she would be thinking, *"What the hell do you know about anything?!"*

But shockingly she was receptive of my ideas and thinking! We connected and in my world, connections meant *everything*. Once you were able to connect with someone you might care for them a little more, you might remember them a little better. Not just in healthcare but anywhere in life. A person is a person. You may know their name or what they do, but until you both connect to each other on some level, there is no depth to your acquaintance. I think I made a new friend in Luna. I put that little personal triumph in my back pocket and would remember it when I went back to check up on her again. I needed to stick her for her 2100 blood sugar and then administer her long-lasting insulin. My 1700 was done by 1730. I sat down and relaxed for a good half hour. I had never been done this early with my med-pass. I was shocked.

I took a look at Luna's chart and saw a plethora of diagnoses. I feared that if she contracted the 'Rona, her recovery might be quite difficult. Towards the end of her admitting diagnoses I saw a diagnosis of "Corona virus." The paper had been printed in January. Maybe she'd brought the COVID here?! I flipped through all the doctor's notes and read somewhere that it wasn't the COVID-19, but an earlier mutation that was still considered a Corona virus. Apparently there were seven different kinds and they were all within a SARS umbrella virus or description. I had much to learn about respiratory viruses. I wondered if Luna could have immunity due to her previous exposure to a different strain.

When I got back to Luna's room that night I decided to let her in on my secrets of sobriety and alcoholism. I walked in to find Luna helping her roommate organize some things on her TV stand/dresser and it hit me on the head like a hammer! I would tell her all about my sobriety and how I was staying sober and what helped to maintain a healthy spiritual life. To this point I had never had the obsession to pick up a drink but did in fact embellish the daily "struggle" of staying sober, when speaking with her. I told her about my bracelet and what it meant to me. I told her about the meeting where I'd received it. It was full of sober alcoholics who'd remained sober for twenty or thirty years. The audience I spoke in front of probably had a combined four or five hundred years of sobriety. It was an honor to speak in front of them and I shared that with Luna. I focused on the fact that anyone could turn their life around at any moment. She appreciated the sentiment and I thought I saw a bit of pity for me coming from her face as she tilted her head. People always felt bad for alcoholics, when in reality, once alcoholics found sobriety and the fellowship of Alcohol Support Groups, they found the key to life. The Alcohol Support Group was the greatest organization in the world and only a minute fraction of the people on earth would ever get to experience it. It was like winning the lottery.

I asked her a question while I was on my way out; "Do you know what our main principle is that we *have* to practice daily to maintain our sobriety and spiritual fitness?"

"Hmm….I don't know." She was unsure of the answer and embarrassed, but still smiled.

"Service to others!" I shouted enthusiastically and closed the door. If I'd had a mic, I would have dropped it. It was a tremendously awkward exit but I had a good feeling about it and thought there was a good chance she might respond to the pep talk. My life coach/therapist role was really taking off.

I spoke with Mel and we made corny jokes. We heard a great uproar of laughter and yelling from the mammoth 2C central nursing station. I told him to go check it out, knowing it was probably just fun times being had amidst all the misery. I wanted to see what was so funny but refused to leave the unit because of safety. I especially always had to keep an eye on Leslie. Her door was the only one, probably in the whole facility, that had to stay open. If we closed the door for more than half an hour, she would surely get up and fall right on her face. We would have to call her family and the doctor. We would have to do a full work up. We would have to call 911 to bring her to the already taxed and overflowing ER. She would then need a CT scan to rule out brain injury from head trauma.

Mel returned and said they were just being stupid. I didn't ask him to elaborate. I felt like they shouldn't be laughing and having a good time, but simultaneously felt happy for them and their ability to laugh in such a sinister setting.

I finished the rest of the night without incident. The following weeks were more of the same.

Chapter 15

April 19th-May 25th

This too, shall pass - Abraham Lincoln

Life was as good as it could get as a COVID nurse. We had plenty of extra hands and lighter resident assignments. Every day the revolving door of COVID quarantine and quarantine releases kept spinning. There was the occasional readmission to quarantine after a resident had come back to their regular floor. Leanne and Jan tested positive again, after being home for more than a week, and became the first casualties of a repeat quarantine admission.

I was stationed at 2B most of the time, but did have to float to quarantine every once in a while. The nurse Lana from Florida would precede me most days when I worked 2B. She took very good care of all my *grandparents* and seemed like she enjoyed it. She certainly enjoyed the money—all the travelers did. The traveling CNAs were making almost double what I was making as an LPN. COVID or not, I would have taken the travel opportunity if I could have (the asterisk on my nursing license wouldn't allow it). Between Lana and I and a regular overnight nurse, our residents were well fed, well medicated and generally well taken care of. The only loss we had so far was Belle Montagne. Like I said before, her quality of life had been minimal and it was only a matter of time before she crossed to the other side. I wondered if COVID had attacked one of her many diagnoses. Could it have exacerbated her COPD? Or did the COVID attack her already weakened heart with its congestive failure? Maybe it worsened her hypertension. She was obese as well, so it could have been that. Maybe the diabetes ran rampant alongside the COVID. She also had coronary artery disease and hyperlipidemia. She was also constantly dehydrated. Maybe COVID affected all these a little and created a perfect storm of system shutdowns. If I had to choose one disease that was worsened by the virus I would choose the COPD. It just seemed logical that a respiratory virus would make matters worse for an individual who couldn't breathe right to begin with. I thought of the dozens of other residents with just as many diagnoses who had survived. Maybe it was just her time.

At any given time I had anywhere from three to fifteen of my regular residents. They were constantly going down to quarantine and coming back. Tabatha Patterson went down to quarantine during this time and I thought for sure I wouldn't see her again. She was eighty-nine, but her only medical history was a stroke that had rendered her right limbs useless—that, and high cholesterol. She had a fever for a day or two, and then kicked COVID to the curb. I concluded that age had nothing to do with morbidity rates. I also concluded that breathing disorders like COPD would be the ultimate factors. I concluded that as a brand new nurse I shouldn't be concluding anything. This type of speculation was wasted thought and energy. I'd leave it to the scientists and the CDC to come up with the statistics.

I did fall victim to something the press was saying about residents on antacids and repelling the virus. I started looking through charts in my newly found spare time. I checked the residents I knew who'd had no fever or other signs of COVID and had never gone to quarantine. The first chart I checked, the resident took Pepcid every day. The next chart—Pepcid again! My hopes rose alarmingly fast. The next two charts of the residents all had Pepcid as well! Just as I was about to phone the CDC headquarters in Atlanta to confirm the recent discovery, I went to the fifth chart and found that the resident had no history of GERD (heartburn) and was not taking any type of antacid. I hung up the imaginary phone I held in my hand and whispered, "Sorry, CDC. No dice. Stand by." Although I was never really going to call the CDC, if I did find that all the residents who were taking famotidine never had any signs or symptoms of the COVID, I figured I would be obligated to tell *someone*. I checked a bunch of other charts and some had the medication and others didn't. It was about 50% and nothing to write home—or the CDC—about. I could imagine half of America overdosing on Pepcid because of the media's suggestive story. Shame on the press. Again.

I sang with Jim almost daily. I picked more famous classic rock songs and before he started to sing with me he named every artist and title of each song. Billy Joel, Beatles, Rolling Stones, Queen, Bruce Springsteen. We sang a song at the 1700 med-pass and another at the 2100. He enjoyed our duets but you couldn't tell. He never smiled and only spoke in short declarative sentences. I know that other residents and CNAs loved hearing our songs.

I also hummed "Silent Night" loudly with Ruby Vedder almost every night. We made heavenly music together. It got old for me and especially for Tabatha who sometimes would yell, "Oh…would…you…drop it already! It's…not…even…*Christmas*!" I would laugh it off and say things like, "Wow, tough crowd tonight! Good night, New Jersey!" I would tell Tabatha that we weren't taking any requests. Tabatha was always in a foul mood. I would be too if I were living in a nursing home receiving average care and relying on others for any semblance of a decent and independent life. Despite our constant bickering I always prayed for her, that she may find peace in this rotten elder-hotel of misery.

Leslie and Barbara's behavior was completely predictable. Barbara stayed in her bed and muttered incoherent nonsense to herself. She would take her medications most of the time. Leslie would sometimes get frustrated with her roommate's rambling and tell her to shut up. If I was around I would sternly tell Leslie to be nice. Sometimes it worked, sometimes it didn't. Without fail, Leslie would try to get up to walk to the bathroom at least two or three times a night. Most nights I would park my cart outside her door whenever I could. She called me Bruce. When she wasn't talking to me and asking questions, she was yelling about who I was and what I was doing there and asking me to leave. Eventually she contracted the virus and went down to quarantine for a two-week stay until she tested negative. During her quarantine time she fell at least twice. She also accused a CNA from Florida of pushing her to the floor. For some reason the powers that be, suspended the CNA until an investigation was completed. When I heard about this I felt like going down to the Director of Nursing's cozy office and screaming at her about how Leslie was full of these accusations almost daily. She had once accused me of raping her in the shower. She hadn't been in a shower for weeks and if she had been, I wouldn't have been the one washing her!

Leslie came back to 2B with a one-on-one (1:1) monitor. His name was Arnie and he was a marine. She only had an order for 1:1 monitoring during the 3 to 11 p.m. second shift, when her sundowning really took flight. They hired Arnie through a temp agency. He had no experience in healthcare or dealing with the elderly, but was a hero anyway. If he could handle two tours in the middle east, babysitting a senile old woman would be a piece of cake. Arnie looked Indian but was from French Guyana and was a real Godsend. He had long black hair in a ponytail, and a goatee. He was thick and stocky and a touch overweight, but a tank nonetheless. His only job was to sit outside Leslie's room and make sure she wasn't trying to walk. If she was, he would call me and I would try to de-escalate the situation. I eventually asked him, "Hey buddy, if no one is around are you ready to run in there and catch her?"

He wasn't crazy about that idea and said he couldn't touch the residents, but I kept working on him knowing that turning him to this kind of thinking was a definite possibility. Eventually, after a couple of weeks of me hammering home this idea, he said he would catch her if need be. I called him a *got-damn hero* in my best southern accent.

Arnie added a whole new dynamic to the floor. I wasn't sure of his level of faith but decided he had to have something within him because he wasn't just watching Leslie. If he heard a resident yelling for something he would go check on them quick enough to not let Leslie get any ideas. As you left Leslie, you would have to count in your head, *okay she could be positioning herself to get up now. Now she could be dangling one leg over the bed... now two legs. Now her arms are on the railing to get ready to pull. Okay, now she's leaning forward to start the walk of faith. Time to get back to her room!* Eventually, Arnie became a pro. He was getting water for people, helping with food trays here and there, and even answering the phone for me once in a while. We became good friends and keep in touch to this day.

We continued to wonder how cunning and baffling this virus was. How was it spreading—who was spreading it?! More speculative thought led nowhere. I took on the physical therapist's role during this time, for residents who needed it. Lying in bed for even a couple of days had serious detrimental effects on a person's muscles and tissue. I tried to stretch their legs and get them moving a bit in bed. There was only so much I could do. Eventually, their muscles would contract and it would take months of physical therapy to reverse the damage.

We learned more and more about our new travel friends. We learned who could be reliable and hardworking. We learned who would do the bare minimum. We learned who was absolute garbage. The good and the bad were always present no matter where you went or what industry or culture you were looking at. When it comes to people's lives and the care for them, the bad could be especially dangerous in an industry like healthcare. If you were responsible for everything for a resident and you were the only one in the room, the bad became deadly. If a resident couldn't advocate for themselves and was being mistreated there would be no way to alert someone else. I found the true champions and treated them very well. I always thanked them profusely and thanked them for coming. People thought because of my sense of humor and sarcastic wordplay that I was kidding when I thanked them for coming, but I was genuinely grateful that they all came to our rescue.

I had to keep relearning the same old book-cover-judgment lesson and just couldn't get past it. There was a CNA from Louisiana named Bridget, whom you could hear from the 2C mega desk all the way down the football hallway. She was borderline obnoxious but high energy, always running around making fun. I thought for sure I or someone else would have to tell her to chill the fuck out and do her job. I dreaded that day. She turned out to be one of the best CNAs I had *ever* worked with! She was certainly loud but she did the best job. She changed residents two to three times a shift, did it with a smile on her face, never once questioned an order, and never complained. One day her shift had ended and she was walking out the door to the stairwell when she saw me in a room ready to change an extra-large resident; she stopped and yelled to me as if I were across an ocean, "David!? What you doin' in dare right now!?" with her backpack on, ready to walk out the stairwell door.

"I'm about to change Miss Grayson," I replied calmly and quietly, trying to encourage her to heed my tone.

"Uh-uh! Go on, git! Git David! I ain't having dat!" she yelled back at me with increasing volume while putting her bag down and stepping inside the room.

"I got this, don't worry—you can go," I said smiling.

"Git David!" she kept yelling. She was persistent in her insistence so I obeyed her command and thanked her repeatedly. She'd worked hard enough and her shift was over. She'd even clocked out so this was a brief change we could label community service. By the time I got to the door, she was halfway done with the change. It took her less than three minutes for the full change and I thanked her again when she finally left, and she said something about not having the nurses changing diapers. I was so touched she did this for me and didn't know why at first. I reasoned that it was because no one else would have ever stopped and come in, especially off the clock, to help me and the resident. I asked God for ten more of her.

Another CNA, Kelly, did an excellent job all around and, it turns out, she specialized in working with the really difficult residents. Rubin Esquivel was a paranoid schizophrenic, who rarely took his meds. He was wary of every person who walked into his room. He kept multiple urinals on his bed right next to him and wouldn't let anyone empty them for him. He would scream and fight everything and everyone. Staff would have to give up out of fear of spilling the urine all over the bed or getting scratched, kicked, or punched. He rarely bathed and refused to let staff change him. After a couple of days of refusals, you would eventually have to bum-rush him with three to five staff members and bathe him kicking and screaming all the while. Kelly somehow and someway got through to him. Rubin let Kelly take care of him every day she was there. She was some type of schizophrenic whisperer. Whenever a nurse would go in to check on him or give him meds he would repeat, "Kelly baby! Where's Kelly? I only want Kelly, she the only one take care of me. Kelly baby, where are you, Kelly?!"

I thought this was incredible! He was one of the worst residents to have on your assignment. I imitated him in a low Spanish accent, talking to Kelly at the nursing station where no residents could hear. I wasn't poking fun at them, but rather pointing out how incredible his response to Kelly was. I publicly congratulated and thanked her so all could hear what an awesome job she did. She still told me to stop making fun of her man and everyone laughed.

We heard of the parties the traveling nurses and CNAs were having in their hotel rooms. I imagined huge orgies and harems of women dressed in scantily clad scrubs and PPE. Many of them were good looking and I considered whether or not finding strange love and sex in cities far away from home were a type of allure when it came to signing travel contracts. We heard of a travel nurse working for us who was found dead in her hotel room a day or two after not reporting to work. We didn't hear anything else about the situation or cause of death so I still question whether or not the story was made up—the gossip and rumors around the facility were tangible and suffocating.

We saw which nurses would stand up to supervisors and management when receiving an unfair assignment. Most of them took the unfair assignments until it was one too many. They bit their tongue, but just like any human being, they had a breaking point and had to stick up for themselves. I learned how important acceptance was in my life, and how crucial a step and belief it was for me to practice daily if I had any chance to get past adversity and stressful situations. There was a line where one would have to stick up for themselves or point out injustices. As a newly sober new nurse, I was still trying to find this line and walk it finely. For the most part, I did whatever the other nurses and supervisors asked of me. I didn't know enough about the nursing world to object when I thought I might be getting treated unjustly or unfairly or put into unsafe situations. I could only advocate for residents in very simple ways thus far. I observed my fellow nurses who traveled from all over to help us. It was from them how I gained nursing experience and wisdom.

I shared the second floor with Stephanie and Shawna. They became fast friends as well. One day Stephanie approached me at the back end of my forty-yard hallway. She was a saucy, spunky, but sweet southerner with a kind of *"Hush, chile' Momma's got you, baby,"* attitude and dialect.

She lowered her head and looked over the top rims of her glasses beginning fierce eye contact with me.

I didn't know what to expect.

"Someone wants to know if you're single."

I laughed nervously but was flattered. It reminded me of some high school matchmaker bullshit. "No comment," I squeaked out. Stephanie persisted and eventually got an answer out of me. I told her I was in a complicated relationship. Things between Candace and I weren't going so well. She wasn't taking quarantine too well. She would spend all day at home and didn't know what to do with herself. She didn't want to clean or cook or do laundry. I still had to share all the domestic duties 50/50 even though she wasn't working at all and I was working overtime. Stephanie apparently thought this was a good thing because she practically bounced back up the hallway with a skip, happy with the news I gave her. I decided it wasn't her because she was married and a little too old for me. For a second I wondered who it might be. I considered it was Shawna or maybe Lana. I spent a lot of time with both of them and we always shared plenty of laughs. Lana kept touching me and rubbing her body against mine at the med-cart. She would put her leg up as if she wanted me to hold it and bring her in close and spin her around and dip her or something. She had a boyfriend back home so this behavior left me incredibly confused. I turned off any and all thought processes and got back to my duties as caretaker, nurse, water boy, foot rubber, emotional therapist, physical therapist, pep-talker, friend, and grandchild.

During this time I watched a nurse walking out of the building with an incredibly athletic physique. I was immediately attracted to her body and particularly her gluteus maximus. I cursed this PPE for taking away all my butt views. I wondered who it was. I had no idea of who it might be since everyone I interacted with daily was covered in plastic PPE. Some people even wore an extra gown backward under their front gown so their clothes were completely untouchable to lingering COVID droplets. The nurse had bleached blonde hair, and then I realized I knew no one's hair color either. I probably couldn't even identify someone's face after working with them for over a month. I would have to pretend like I was a camera-less photographer trying to plan out a shot of their forehead and eyes, making a rectangle with my thumb and index finger of both hands when looking at a nurse covered head to toe in PPE. One nurse made a funny joke about someone being really into eyes as a physical attribute and how they would have been in heaven cause that was all you saw during PPE COVID wartime (I would retell it but I couldn't do the joke its proper justice). Everyone at the mega 2C desk burst out in laughter after hearing the eye fetish joke.

Road traffic was getting back to normal by now and I found myself riding carelessly on my bike when I should have been paying more attention. I never wore a helmet—but don't tell my mother! I got an adrenaline rush from weaving in and out of traffic— *safely*. The trains were still empty except for a few other health care workers and other essential employees. I liked to think that we shared a kind of, "Yeah, this sucks, we're still here working while everyone else is sitting at home getting paid!" type of silent acknowledgement. I did get a wild thank you from a motorist while riding my bike to work one day. She pulled over so abruptly I thought something was wrong or she was going to yell at me for riding too slow, but I was on the sidewalk! I prepared myself for a confrontation and she yelled at her window, "Thank you for what you're doing!"

I exhaled and yelled back, "YA WELCOME BABY!" She beeped a couple friendly beeps and went on her way. It was a funny interaction and sort of made my day. It was the only recognition I got from the public aside from family and friends seeing me a year after the onset of the pandemic. We watched reports of the people in Italy opening their windows and applauding all the healthcare workers at the change of shift. I believe this became a common occurrence in New York as well and maybe other places. Leave it to Europe to start some cool trend that I would never get to experience.

On the train platform, I also saw my homeless friend hanging out with other transients and he recognized me through the mask and said hello. He would panhandle outside my gym and we arranged that I would give him five dollars a week to watch my bike while it was locked in the gym lobby. I had already had my last bike stolen on a busy main street in my city. Weeks later I saw someone trying to cut my new bike lock cut off my new bike and caught him in the action. He was a big guy for a thief, but my Alcohol Support Groups friend and I scared him off. My homeless friend was happy with his allowance and agreed to watch the bike, though I doubt he ever did. He was too busy greeting pedestrians and asking them for money.

At this point, the virus was still very scary so I'm not sure if it was because he didn't want to get near me in my scrubs or because he was just caught off guard, but he didn't ask me for any money that day. I hadn't seen him in over two months and in that same time I'd started my career as a nurse. He only knew me as a fitness freak with a bandana and earbuds riding my bike. He knew I was often going to and from meetings and I always invited him but his need for money kept him from attending a meeting with me. He was an addict currently taking Suboxone but was apparently clean and going to Addict Support Group (the sister fellowship of Alcohol Support Group) meetings on his own time. He told me he had a degree in accounting from a local university. We were completely opposite but entirely the same. We were the same person at different points in our lives. I had a roof over my head and a good job, he was panhandling the streets, but we both shared addiction and recovery and that connection meant *everything*.

Shawna, Stephanie, and I worked the 2ⁿᵈ floor like clockwork. The fourth post was usually a random traveler or regular facility nurse. Between the three of us, our residents continued to get excellent care. They came to me when they had general questions about residents or were trying to locate supplies. I helped them for the first couple of weeks but once they got the lay of the land I was the one coming to them for help and advice. We always had sit-down time even after all the vital signs and medication. We would surprise each other with coffees, candies, and energy drinks.

Up to this point, I had only been a nurse for three months and more than half of that was during COVID. I was constantly rattled and overwhelmed. I was taking care of my residents, but for the most part, I was stressed and my behavior and interactions with residents often showed it. I could be very short with residents on top of having a very short fuse. I watched as Shawna and Stephanie interacted with each resident. They genuinely cared for each resident as if they were family. It amazed me and I decided I had to approach each resident like that. Since we were their only contact, we had to make it extra special. Shawna and Stephanie did all the little things too. I know I occasionally sang and made jokes, but *their* demeanor was genuine and they truly cared for the residents they'd known less than a month. Something about their love and emotion made it really sweet and the residents adored them, especially with their cuddly southern accents.   Outside the resident rooms, we chatted and made jokes and talked about our past lives. Stephanie eluded to a particularly scandalous past of Shawna's. Eventually, Shawna came out and admitted to being an exotic dancer. Shawna had an amazing body and I eventually found out that she was the one I'd seen in the parking lot from behind. She also had an amazing personality and was fun to be around. All the staff took a shine to her in addition to her residents. CNAs and other nurses walked from the other side of the floor to sit and hang out for ten minutes, hoping her southern charm and effervescent personality would rub off on them. She had funny and interesting stories and if staff were lucky enough, they might get to hear some of them. She was from Texas and Louisiana. She and Bridget called themselves the *Louisianimals*. Most of the travelers were fun and exciting and on top of all that, and *much more* importantly, they kicked ass at their job.

Chapter 16

May 26-July 1st

Be the change you want to see in the world - Mahatma Gandhi

I had no cable at home so I had absolutely no connection to current events. Even if I did have cable I wouldn't be caught watching CNN or any other news station, *especially* now with nothing but COVID airing and the endless speculation and fear-mongering. I was in Winston Wheeler's room when I saw scenes of thousands of protestors in the streets. I watched in awe—*What the fuck!? These types of things will completely undo any progress we may have accomplished through lockdowns over the past two months.* I kept watching with Winston. He kept looking at me and then the TV as if to say, "Hey, bro, you gotta get back to work and get out of my room."

I learned the story of George Floyd and how his life had been taken by a police officer in Minnesota. They showed some footage and stated how the officer had been kneeling on his neck for more than ten minutes. They showed onlookers and captioned what they were saying. My heart hurt and I felt uneasiness in my stomach. Just what our country needed in the middle of this stupid fucking pandemic. Our country was literally burning and I was trapped in this geriatric jailhouse watching bits and pieces of the coverage while going in and out of each room.

Surprisingly there wasn't too much chatter about the murder. We worked with a lot of African-Americans so I thought the issue might be talked about non-stop. From what I heard from most of the African-Americans, they had a sense of practical disbelief. They were shaming the officer, but knew it was a common occurrence. They named other people who had died in similar manners. None were too shocked by the tragedy since it happened regularly. I was sad for them, but understood their mentality and position.

I guess since no one in the country was working, they were able to attend the protests and boy, oh boy, did they! Streets in every city across the country were filled with protestors. Social media and its celebrities went nuts posting memes and tweeting anti-racist rants.

I thought about the good versus bad in society. I believed that the good would always prevail, but in some industries, a tiny bit of bad could cost lives. In healthcare when the bad were responsible for the lives of the disabled it could become very dangerous, especially when no one was around. The same theme was present in law enforcement. Give a bad man a gun and a badge, and danger and death would be right around the corner. I tried not to judge anyone including the officer because it simply wasn't my place, but I thought about how much power, responsibility and opportunity people could have and if that person wasn't mentally and spiritually fit, bad things could happen. I prayed for the officer's soul and especially George Floyd's and his grieving family. I prayed for the entire country and hoped we might find peace and resolution.

Winston Wheeler had suffered a stroke about four months before and I had taken care of him before during my orientation. Recently, he moved to our floor. Because of his hemiplegia he could not use the left side of his body. He was especially kind to everyone but could get very agitated very quickly. He had aphasia (unable to express thoughts into words). He could take information and understand what you were saying or needed, but in terms of responding all he could say was *yes, no,* and *yeah!* When we brought him speech tools and letter boards to point out letters and make words, he didn't even want to try. I found out from his wife in February (before COVID) that he was some sort of minister in a local Church and also did some marriage counseling. I tried to pray with him when I could. I only ever said The Lord's Prayer in front of him. I thought he would be excited and delighted to be able to pray with someone, but he never seemed too enthusiastic. I attributed that to the brain damage he'd suffered months before. I talked to his wife and she thought praying with him was a good idea. I never prayed as much as I could have with him. I watched TV with him and he laughed a scared laugh when the news was on, reporting the racial and civil injustices.

During this time, once the general public was allowed out of their houses, his wife started showing up daily. She would come to his window and wave to everyone who could see her. She told the staff how she prayed for her husband every day and how she also included all the other residents and staff in her prayers. I was grateful that I was in her prayers and I put her in mine as well. We needed all the prayer we could get. When she saw a staff member come to the window she would wave and then repeatedly bow a low and long bow. She would then wave with both hands and then make fists and raise them up and down in a sign of victory and inspiration. I started to tear up when I saw her triumphant gestures *every single night*. I still get teary-eyed when I think of the daily faith she exhibited, and her complete devotion to her husband and his recovery. She would call my unit and I would get Winston the portable phone, put it on speaker, and then move him towards the window so he could see his wife while talking to her. They would do their best to try and converse but it was always a one-sided conversation. It was mainly Winston's wife saying prayers and jokingly telling him to behave. He would weep every day during his wife's visits. Despite all the terrible things happening, she embodied true faith and hope and everyone was touched and inspired by her visits. She missed one day because of car trouble but otherwise, she kept it up for almost six months, like clockwork. *Every single day.*

I went to bed one night after caring for Winston and waving to his wife and getting them on the phone together. As I lay in bed I remembered his urinal sitting on his bedside table next to his dinner tray. I had forgotten to empty it. I figured he must have eaten his dinner with the half-full urinal right next to his dinner tray. I felt terrible about forgetting to empty it. I had no choice but to accept that I had failed Winston and his wife. I was human after all, and I had to do my best to let it go. I figured that my batting average was still pretty high in regards to urinal emptying and that no one ever bats a thousand forever...

For how intense the outside was getting, I would have expected more conversation regarding George Floyd amongst coworkers, but I guess we were all on the same page. I don't think I ever heard someone say that the officer's actions were justified. I guess everyone agreed that it was a terrible tragedy that could have been avoided. I heard a couple of CNAs talking about going to a protest in NYC on their day off. I'm not sure if those two ever made it but I know a handful went to a couple of different protests and I was happy for them. They contributed to one of the largest social movements since the civil rights movement of the 1960s. As a white man, I wasn't sure I'd be welcome to join a predominantly African-American protest. I never even considered it. I thought maybe they'd think it wasn't my fight. Maybe they would think I was part of the problem. On TV I saw some white supporters here and there, but decided not to go. I could pray for them from afar.

A couple weeks later we learned of Brianna Taylor and the no-knock warrant from police who showed up at the wrong house. She was an EMT. This particularly resonated with me because police, firemen, EMTs and nurses all shared a certain type of professional respect for each other. She probably wasn't in her EMT uniform sitting at home—did that mean they thought she was no good because she was black? It scared me to think of these things and the possibilities out there in this crazy new world. I felt like we needed to go back into a strict lockdown until we could all get ourselves right.

During this time there were no gyms for physical outlets and stress release. Doctor's offices were closed so people couldn't see their therapists for mental and emotional support. All my meetings were closed so I couldn't get the in-person support I needed as a sober alcoholic. Places of worship were closed so spiritual refreshment wasn't available to regular churchgoers either. People were getting squirrelly at an alarming rate. I hoped we as a nation and a civilization would get better… and fast. All I could do was focus on my residents and getting to work each day. In order to help change the world, I had to focus on my small community and make a difference here, before anything else could happen. I heard one of Mahatma Gandhi's most famous quotes in my head: "Be the change you want to see in the world."

I decided to really help Luna Wolfe in any way I could. I wanted to pull her out of her abyss of despair and self-pity. Where would I start? I started by listening. I was always great at listening to people. I never waited to talk and boasted a 86% retention rate of what people told me. I didn't have actual statistics but I retained a lot of what people said because I usually did care, and had an enormous amount of compassion and empathy, which could sometimes get me in trouble. Luna went on about how unfair it was to be living in a nursing home at the age of fifty-nine. She stated how she didn't understand how she could be in such a situation. She was recently diagnosed with multiple sclerosis and maybe hadn't accepted it yet. She'd also been diagnosed with Diabetes since her hospital admission and stated how she'd always had her hemoglobin A1C tested and it had never shown her to be a diabetic—not even pre-diabetic! She also had chronic kidney disease. The gloom and doom surrounded and drowned her.

One day while prancing around Luna's room waiting for her blood pressure to read, I noticed she had a book about George R.R. Martin and how the Fire and Ice books were written—common ground! We could connect and I could change the subject! We started talking about the books and refused to mention the HBO show at all. I had read three of the books during my two-month stay at the county jail. My wonderful mother sent me all five books while I was locked up with other alcoholics and heroin addicts-turned thieves. Reading kept me sane while my freedom was taken from me. I shared this with her and told her I knew exactly how it felt to be locked up in a room with no liberties.

For some reason, I kept telling her stories about my alcoholism and my ongoing journey through it. I felt I could trust her even though I had only known her for a month and our friendship wasn't that deep. The other alcoholics in my Alcohol Support Groups always said to maintain your anonymity and tell no one about your sobriety for a variety of reasons which I won't get into. I'd always been open with my life and my shortcomings and decided the misery I'd endured might help Miss Wolf in some sort of way. I was proud of my sobriety and the adversity I'd overcome, and kept believing that she would benefit from hearing my alcoholic tales.

She was also a good listener and was immediately entranced by the trials and tribulations I'd gone through. I told her how every day I practiced gratitude and how I always thought about my situation being worse. I wanted her to know I truly believed in the "It could always be worse," attitude. I told her how I could have been addicted to heroin or I could have been crippled in one of my many drunk driving accidents. I told her how it was a miracle I wasn't in jail for the rest of my life for drinking and driving and potentially killing an innocent person. Maybe it was at this point in time where she changed her thinking. Maybe it was because she thought we might be friends. It could have been the common ground we found in literature-especially sci-fi/fantasy novels. Maybe it was all of the above. Maybe it was just me but she seemed to be in a better mood since that day I opened up to her.

I hopped around room to room doing what I could and exuding an "I really care" approach I'd recently learned from Shawna and Stephanie. I guess it was more about having a little experience under my belt and having less residents, that I had time for heart-felt, genuine interactions with my residents, but Stephanie and Shawna certainly helped enlighten me to the importance of showing real love to our residents. More and more residents were surviving the death sentence that came with the COVID diagnosis and were coming back to our floor. By this time, only one or two would go to quarantine each week and three or four would return! Everyone was making it back. Mostly everyone. Because I knew the nurses were swamped on the COVID units, I still never called to check up on my people and left it up to God to decide my residents' fates. After working with all these residents I really did feel responsible for them and felt connected to them. If my residents were happy and healthy I was doing a good job. If they were sick and unhappy I felt like a failure and considered what I might do better for each of them individually.

I continued to get to know Shawna and Stephanie and kept observing their practice and learning how to be a good nurse. I learned that Shawna was single and might or might not be interested in me. Stephanie gave me hints as to her interest and I wondered if Shawna was the one Stephanie had been talking about when she'd asked about my romantic status. Shawna and I flirted at the nurse's station most of the time we worked together. We shared a love for physical fitness and working out. I hadn't always loved the gym because I'd always been too busy drinking, but since I got sober it was something I did six days a week and was one of my most time-consuming hobbies. I liked the way I looked after working out for nearly two years, but I did it mainly for my mental health. Whenever I got a gym day in, I was mentally and emotionally on cloud nine. If I made an Alcohol Support Group meeting that same day, forget about it! I was living in complete and utter ecstasy.

Shawna and I talked about favorite exercises and gym etiquette and how exercise made us feel. We poked playful fun at the gym-goers who would show up for a week and do the silliest of exercises, only to never be seen again. We talked about how these same people would move all the equipment and weights around into funny arrangements, do one set and then leave all the equipment scattered in the middle of the floor. The old me would get angry and rush to judge these morons in the gym but since Alcohol Support Groups taught me new ways of thinking, I decided to change my attitude towards them and their efforts. I decided I should be happy that they were at the gym and trying at all! One of them might keep coming back and find out that if they work it, it works!

We commiserated about how gyms were closed and how we weren't particularly fond of body weight exercises and calisthenics. We preferred to pump iron and tons of it over and over again. One night the police officer turned nurse—Blake—jumped in and told us about his medicine balls and squats. Shawna and he talked about squatting. I got jealous and wanted to tell him to back off—but I had to eradicate my selfish self-seeking behavior driven by my small but ever-present ego. I laughed it off after I learned he was married with a child at home. I thought of Candace at home and how I was being doubly selfish. Shawna was well-liked and extremely popular so I had to share her attention with everyone else who came for a conversation with her. The PPE rules had become a little more lax and nurses didn't wear the heavy plastic gowns at nursing stations anymore. We decided that being cool and comfortable was more important than tiny droplets coming into contact with our scrubs, (the goggles and N95 were still mandatory and would protect our mucous membranes and respiratory tracts) which we would carefully handle after our shift and then wash. I saw Shawna's butt all the time and was mesmerized. I wasn't the only one who was looking though. All the male residents were also entranced. All the staff who were comfortable enough with her complimented her on her round and perfect rump. Bridget and other CNAs constantly commented on how perfect and large it was for a white girl. Bridget even went as far as slapping it regularly, but Shawna enjoyed the attention. Shawna continued to show interest in me and we eventually went on a day date to Ideal Beach on a Monday that we both had off. I lied to Candace and said I was out doing something else. I felt terrible for deceiving Candace, but felt alive when I was with Shawna. That day and the following week, I struggled with the mixed emotions of euphoria during the honeymoon phase of a new relationship and the impending doom and heartbreak that would accompany breaking up with Candace and the guilt I would feel. You could see Manhattan from Ideal Beach and they even had Alcohol Support Groups every evening around 5:30, right on the beach. Things were really looking up and me and Shawna kissed on the beach. She looked great in a bathing suit too and was very laid back and easy to get along with.

I had an overwhelming feeling of gratitude on the beach that day. I couldn't help but to think of what COVID had brought me. A new romance. One month of hazard pay. Two $1,500 retention bonuses. New friends from all around the country. And most importantly, the opportunity to really make a difference in these residents' lives. I also had to acknowledge the skills and strategies I'd learned from real crisis nurses. I felt like God laid out my path, threw me on it, and watched me blossom into the man I was destined to become. God carried me to the biggest and most pivotal moments of my life. It was like His plan for my growth was completed moments before worldwide anarchy and chaos would erupt. I was primed and ready to be a real man just in time for the COVID pandemic. After surviving and thriving on the frontlines of COVID I was sure I could handle anything, and maybe I could confidently call myself a real nurse after the first four months of absolute turmoil. I considered that maybe four months of pandemic nursing was actually equivalent to two regular years of nursing.

At this juncture, our death toll was in the double digits, somewhere around sixteen. We never told the other residents of the deaths piling up. We tried to keep it light and fun as best we could. In addition to my nursing I continued to try to entertain residents. Since the recreation department was still on leave, the residents had nothing to do except watch the news, eat, sleep and take their pills. I was the only entertainment they had. I came up with new material and new songs in my spare time. Many of my residents were on the drug Gabapentin for nerve pain and neuropathy. The residents who did receive it got it three to four times a day, every four to six hours while awake. I sang a song for those customers as I gave it to them:

Gabapentin in the morning,

Gabapentin in the evening,
Gabapentin at supper time,
When gabapentin's in a capsule,
You can have gabapentin any time!

I would look up jokes before my shift to tell the residents in their rooms in hopes that a laugh or two would get them through the day. Sometimes I would get distracted and forget my material. Other times the jokes wouldn't land, and occasionally I would get a great laugh from some residents. My new job as comedian in the nursing home was perfect because I never had to worry about coming up with new material. Most of the residents would forget the jokes I told the day before. I told them about my beautiful library and how a book fell on my head and how I had only my *shelf* to blame. Some understood that joke, others didn't. No matter what, Tabatha Patterson would roll her eyes and tell me my stuff wasn't funny.

For Leslie Dawson I would sing Barry Manilow's song "Copa cabana":

Her name was Leslie,
She was a showgirl,
With a bow up in her hair,
Her gown was cut to there,
She would merengue,
And do the cha-cha
And while she tried to watch TV,
She would always hide from me,
Across your room, I'm here,
Not going nowhere!
We're young and we have each other!
Who could ask for more!
AT THE COVID! COVID CABANA!
The hottest spot north of Corona!

I started rolling my arms and fists like John Travolta in Saturday Night Fever while attempting to move my feet in a salsa dance-type way. She loved it and smiled ear to ear. I kept singing this song to Leslie (and Arnie the marine) until I found out she loved the Beatles. I sang all the Beatles songs I knew but it didn't tickle her as much. She would sometimes say I was off-key or flat or she'd just ask me to shut up. I tried not to take offense and let it slide. I deemed her confused because my singing was always pitch-perfect. Her roommate Barbara got "Barbara Ann" from the Beach Boys, but the only part I knew was the main chorus and the "Rocking and a rolling," but Barbara enjoyed it just the same. She responded with an excited smile and her classic, "Aight!"

The Alcohol Support Group's zoom meetings were still going strong. More meetings kept opening up online and newly sober alcoholics could find the help they needed. The need to help other alcoholics achieve sobriety was an ever-present practice we engaged in to maintain our sobriety. When I was six months sober I was asked to join Alcohol Support Group's "Night Watch." It was funny because The Night's Watch from George R.R. Martin's "A Song of Fire and Ice" never got involved in the realm's politics or issues. Their only mission was to guard the wall from the wildlings. In my Alcohol Support Groups we had a similar practice. We would stay out of politics and current events and would receive no financial support from any establishments or institutions and especially corporate organizations. This would keep us free from outside influence and enable us to focus on our mission to stay sober and help others do the same. We were a self-run and self-supported organization of anonymity. The Night's Watch from the novels and my Night Watch from my Alcohol Support Groups shared practically the same name and the same primary belief. Night Watch was a program for alcoholics in crisis. They would call our number and be routed to an Alcohol Support Group member who had signed up to be on call. During my first two years on the list of Night Watch I never received a single phone call. Within the first three months of the pandemic I had fielded three phone calls of alcoholics in crisis. I listened as best I could and told them what worked for me. I was careful to never give advice. I told them to get the free ZOOM application and start attending online meetings. This rise in phone calls was no doubt due to COVID. I pictured alcoholics drinking all day every day at home in complete darkness and misery—a scene I knew all too well. I wished I could save them all. The truth was that even the ones who did want be saved and did ask for help would still have difficulty with getting sober.

It was no cakewalk in the park. Regardless of the uphill task, we, as sober alcoholics, heard the call and had to be eager to help every time, even if the case seemed hopeless. Even after you tried to help thirty people and they *all* went back to drinking, you had to keep helping others and show them what sobriety could do for them. I shared these comparisons to Game of Thrones with Luna and emphasized the important practice of service to others, in hopes I would hammer home the idea. I wanted her to know I wasn't just all talk. I was practicing service to others daily, not just as a paid nurse, but also as a sober alcoholic giving back what had been freely given to me. I told her how Daft Punk always told me that *work is never over.*

By the end of June, I estimated nearly 70% of our residents had had the virus at one point and the majority had survived. I estimated that out of about 170 residents, a hundred residents had been in and out of quarantine and the death toll was in the low 20s. This was a mortality rate of about 15%, which was much higher than the survival rate of the population outside of the nursing home. As I mentioned earlier, many of these residents had multiple diagnoses that complicated the COVID. Many of them were in their seventies and eighties. Many of them were already completely debilitated to the point where they never left their bed, so it was no wonder our morbidity percentages were much higher than those of the outside world. I'll mention again the fact that we had handfuls of residents into their nineties surviving the COVID.

Sometime during June we heard rumors of the isolation and quarantine ending. At the end of June or the beginning of July, residents were allowed to be outside their rooms while wearing surgical masks. We were about to enter PHASE 2 of the governor's plan for reopening with strict sanctions and requirements. The light at the end of the tunnel could be seen…

Chapter 17

July 2ⁿᵈ -August 30ᵗʰ

Time takes time - Unknown

The governor reopened the state with plenty of restrictions and sanctions, but regardless of the new norms being imposed, the masses rejoiced. There was no indoor dining so restaurants took to the streets and parking lots and any unoccupied spaces to put tents and tables for their patrons to return. Gyms were still not open but it was a start. Time takes time. This is what the 'old-timers' told newcomers in the Alcohol Support Groups who wanted their sobriety fast. Sometimes newcomers would wish for ten years of sobriety overnight. They wished to be able to be around alcohol safely or to get rid of the urges or ideas of drinking, in an instant. They wanted to be free of drunk dreams. They wanted what they wanted and they wanted it right away. "Time takes time" was a widely used slogan in circles of recovery and it often accompanied the "One day at a time" motto. In the pandemic wartime, we had to take it slow and safe in order to get back to normal, healthy living.

In the nursing home, residents were allowed outside of their rooms for the first time in over three months. The residents still had to wear masks, but for this elderly and confused population we had to constantly remind them or send them back to their rooms if they didn't comply. Dwayne Johnson's The Rock persona rang loudly in my head, "Finallyyyyy, The hot corner!…Has come back!…To Norwich!" The hot corner was back and buzzing, baby! I was excited as all get-out!

I came back after a weekend off to find Lucie Greer, Tabatha Patterson,

Anita Gregg, Leslie Dawson, Wally Lasiter, and a few others lined up at the hall sitting and talking. Tabatha kept going on about how terrible it was and how unfair it had gotten towards the end. People were getting back into their wheelchairs and out of their lonely isolation. It was a happy sight and I told them how glad I was to see them out and about. They were unable to eat in the dining room, but they were happy with the slight progress this new freedom brought them. I had heard of everyone being allowed outside of their rooms and considered that maybe the residents would be too afraid of getting sick again and wouldn't want to. I came through the stairwell door and when I saw them all sitting there I got the idea for a funny bit:

"OH. MY. GAWD!" I slowed down to stop while I spoke like Janice from "Friends," looking around cautiously as I did.

The residents all looked at me and at each other and then at the other staff. Even the CNAs and other nurse were confused. I put my hands together and looked up at the ceiling and then back to each one of them, keeping my Janice imitation going, "You guys remembered! My birthday!" I started running and jumping in place over-excitedly. "Oh my gosh, this is incredible! Thank you so much!"

The hot corner exploded with laughter. Lucie and Wally laughed because they understood the joke. Anita laughed because of the physical comedy. Leslie laughed because the others were laughing. Jordan didn't laugh, just rolled his eyes, but I could tell he was entertained because he continued to watch my every move. The staff watching my bit understood the joke and thought it was funny as well. Of course, Tabatha laughed out of sympathy thinking I was foolish, but she was also annoyed at everyone's laughter at my joke.

"We're... not... celebrating... your birthday!" She acted as if she was breaking sad news to me while also yelling at me for leaving some door open somewhere.

"Wait. What?" I said quietly. I lowered my head and pretended to realize I had gotten it all wrong, "Oh man. I thought you guys organized this whole thing for me..." I started to walk back to the desk lowering my head and as I did I yelled, "My mother was right! I am an *idiot!*"

The whole corner exploded with laughter again. After such a positive response from the crowd, I decided right then and there that entertaining these folks and making them laugh was just as important as giving them their silly medications. I figured that fella Patch Adams was on to something. I thought about how comedy always made me feel better and how when I first got sober, watching stand-up comedians made me feel great.

It wasn't all fun and games though. It was a pandemic lull during this time, but a pandemic nevertheless. Things were better, but everyone still had to be cautious and stay wary of the COVID.

Tanya was sitting at the desk and commented on my bit and then immediately got serious and stated glumly, "Adrian passed away over the weekend."

"Damn. From what? Covid?" I asked sadly while thinking about whether my birthday surprise bit was insensitive. Most of these residents knew Adrian and the way he yelled from his room. None of the hot corner had a friendship with Adrian, but they were still neighbors. I decided that most of these residents were used to their neighbors passing away—after all, nursing homes were life's end zone. Especially after COVID, they were used to learning of deaths. They had already lost their neighbor Belle Montagne a month before.

Tanya then filled me in on how Adrian had passed due to septicemia, or sepsis. His craterous wound on his buttocks had finally gotten infected and had spread through his bloodstream. I guessed that he succumbed to an infection a week or two before and it eventually caused a total shutdown. He was a DNR and DNI so we wouldn't send him out to a hospital for treatment. The local hospitals were still busy, so the fact that they didn't have to take care of non-compliant combative residents like Adrian because of his code status, was a plus. I prayed that his soul was at rest and hoped that he crossed over peacefully. He taught me valuable lessons about preparation and persistence and reminded me of the importance of patience.

Now that residents were back outside the rooms I had to watch for hazards on the floor. Every mealtime brought hot water and coffee on the floor from careless CNAs pouring the hot beverages from the large carafes and dripping them everywhere. I made it a habit of keeping one eye on the floor for spills and my other eye on the ceiling looking for call bells ringing—head on a swivel—always alert and observing. Elopement was another thing we didn't have to worry about during quarantine, so now we also had to keep an eye on residents who liked to wander and try and escape. Some didn't try to escape, but would go into other residents' rooms and steal things or torment the inhabitants. Even with the extra work, I was happy they were coming out of their forced hermit lifestyles.

Everyone was growing their hair and beards out and I was no exception. I shaved my head into a mohawk and eventually into a long and glorious mullet. With all the masks and head gear I also took advantage of growing a burly mountain man beard. I considered some facial piercings but knew my mother would be upset and decided against it.

Some of the traveling workers had already left, but the rest still had a couple of weeks on their three-month contracts, and many of them were asked to stay on for an additional three months.

Shawna and Stephanie signed on for another three months. Mel, Bridget, and Kelly also stayed on to "...get that COVID money." The rates they were receiving dropped a little bit but this kind of money was still a once-in-a-lifetime opportunity, so most of the travelers stuck around to cash in and continue to make a difference. CNAs and nurses were paying off auto loans, school loans, putting down payments on houses, and starting their own businesses. I was happy they were able to better their lives with the funds. Aside from the one month of hazard pay and two $1,500 retention bonuses we didn't really get anything else except for a month-and-a-half of free food. I did feel like I was bettering my career by working with all the experienced nurses and CNAs. I'd also found Shawna and knew she was made for me. We hung out at least weekly and I even started to stay at her hotel room a couple of nights a week. I broke up with Candace on July 28th and felt terrible about it. The guilt consumed me and I found it very difficult to enjoy the new relationship forming with Shawna. In addition to the break up of the old and the euphoria of the new, I realized this was the first adult relationship that ended with me sober. My emotions were extra sensitive because my body was free of the numbing agents they had gotten so used to.

I moved out of our apartment and back into my sister and brother-in-law's basement. I'd lived there for exactly a year when I'd first gotten sober. They loved having me back. I was the dog walker, the dishwasher, the house sitter, the security guard, the laundry attendant, and the company for my sister when her husband was out of town on business. My thoughts were monopolized by Candace and the trauma I brought to her, but I knew it was the right decision. If I continued a relationship with her while doubting every second of it and not loving her with all my heart, it would be unfair to her. I hoped she would understand this one day. She was a great person and a great girlfriend, but she just wasn't for me. If I had stayed with her, I would have settled, knowing that there could have been a better match out there for me as well as for her. I couldn't live a life full of regret, uncertainty, and what-ifs. What I had with Shawna was everything fairy tales and love stories were made of. The physical attraction was there and the chemistry was almost palpable. We shared many of the same views and philosophies about living life. We were outlaws and rule-breakers who finally got it together enough to have a legitimate career and impact on the world around us. We'd changed most of our ways, but parts of the old us still remained ingrained in the old layers beneath our new ones- we still enjoyed bending the rules.

My sister and brother-in-law bought another house in our hometown thirty minutes south. Since I was living with them in their first house, I helped them pack and move all their stuff little by little. The new house came with a pool, so once they were finally moved in I spent a lot of time over there during the summer. Soon I introduced Shawna to a couple of family members who were there swimming. Everyone was intrigued and entranced by my southern belle. They knew I'd broken up with Candace, but hadn't known about Shawna. Given my historically erratic and eccentric behavior and personality and my imperfect and often hectic life, bringing a new girlfriend to a family function weeks after a major breakup wasn't exactly shocking to them. They all asked the same questions about whether or not Shawna was "carrying." Shawna told everyone that that was the first thing I'd asked her when I'd learned of her Texan origins. Everyone asked us how it was on the frontlines and how we were holding up. We answered the best we could.

I told them how the travelers were so fun and worked so hard and how all these residents were getting the best care while in their hands. I told them about how much I was learning from everyone, especially Shawna and Stephanie. I told them about Evelyn and all the other come-back kids. I tried to name all the ninety-year-old-plus residents who beat COVID and came back to us. They couldn't believe those stories. By this time the world had learned that COVID wasn't a death sentence and the pandemic wouldn't wipe out a third of the population like the plagues hundreds of years before. I continued to spread the good news. I encouraged my family to share the success stories as well. I wanted everyone in the world to know that we were winning the war on COVID. Any COVID front line was ugly and gruesome, but the silver linings were large and shiny and just needed some uncovering. Pandemic or no pandemic, life would go on. It *had* to!

The *Black Lives Matter* movement was still roaring. I remember seeing scenes of officers kneeling alongside protestors and how shocked I was to see that. In this single act, the officers deflated their entire ego, which is practically impossible for most people to do, and showed the protestors true compassion. That was the epitome of taking the high road and showing the protestors that they understood and wanted to help. The good and the bad. One bad apple could ruin an entire profession's reputation and public perception.

Protestors and organizations called for the defunding and disassembling of police departments everywhere. I understood completely the outrage the minority protestors felt but I could not support a nation where there were no police. I thought of complete anarchy. It would be a world where we would police ourselves—what a vision! I joked with everyone about how I never got along with cops, but how I hated the thought of anarchy without them. There would be no consequences for a crime so anything would go and that was a scary thought! Videos of police circulated on the web and social media, of good deeds they were doing. Buying birthday cakes for families that couldn't afford them. Buying shoes for homeless folks. Providing an escort or giving a ride to someone in need. All this positive publicity didn't do much for the folks calling for the disenfranchisement of the police departments, but they needed all the good press they could get. Portland went as far as to occupy a section near city hall and the police department let them have it and sit there for months. What the heck was going on?! We hardly talked about it at work and if we did, everyone shared the same view that what happened in Minnesota was cold-blooded murder, and that was it. I prayed for my nation and hoped it would get back on its feet and we could coexist peacefully. We had the COVID that was dying down, the civil rights movement that was going strong, and a historic and unprecedented presidential race coming up. Our country needed to heal in every sense of the word and in every aspect of our lives. I was certainly not getting involved in the civil rights movement, I was front-line COVID and that was my calling for the moment; anything more might upset the delicate balance I had to maintain to keep my sobriety.

I turned my attention to Luna Wolfe and decided I had to get her out of bed and give her a sense of purpose. She told me stories of how she used to do a lot of community service. She worked with literacy organizations that brought books to children and taught them how to read. She told me how she used to help out the less fortunate and the homeless. She also loved working with animals. Due to her love of mankind and the fact that we had no animals to tend to, I decided that she would need to help some suffering souls around the facility. This would give her that sense of purpose and reason to get out of bed each day.

I discussed this with her and I could tell that she was open to the idea, but wasn't exactly doing cartwheels. I had already planted the seed a couple of weeks before when I'd told her about "service to others" during a goosebumps walk away—as if she'd never heard of service to others! In order for myself and my comrades in my Alcohol Support Groups to stay sober, the first thing we did was help others get sober. We would help the new alcoholic in any way we could. We would make phone calls, make meetings with them, hang out and listen when they just needed company. This type of service meant the world to the alcoholic hoping to stay sober. Service to others was everything to us and anyone else who wanted to live a happy and full life. I told her that maybe she wouldn't live here forever, but for the time being, she could help as many people around here as she could handle; and there were plenty of people who needed help. "Faith without works is dead," I told Luna after our discussion ended and I walked out. I hoped Luna would see the light and hear a calling. I was hoping for another goosebumps walk away/mic drop, but gave up hope. I assumed she would think I was young, dumb, and naive, and that after a long life lived there was no more time or energy for this type of thing and one could do nothing but look after themselves...

When I returned that night at 21:00 for her nightly insulin she asked me what she could do and who needed help. I told her I had no idea where to start or who to start with, but that there were plenty of people who needed help. I pondered on this for a little bit and then figured that a good place to start was exercise, which would also be beneficial to her, her diabetes, and her obesity.

We generally had anywhere from five to ten customers at the hot corner each day just sitting and talking. I told her she could lead exercises for all of them, and how important it would be to get their bodies back to moving and their blood flowing. I told her how much everyone had regressed physically and how important it was for them to get exercise. Through this group exercise, they would also get plenty of social interaction as well. Luna was nervous, but there was also a champion underneath all her sorrow, pain, and self-pity. So she started the very next day.

Her mortal enemy was Tabatha, and Tabatha was not having any of it. Everyone else responded well and started doing fifty arm raises, left then right. Fifty front kicks, both legs. Fifty punches each arm. After a while, Tabatha saw everyone else participating and that led her to join in because she looked odd just sitting and looking on, not doing anything, although she could only do her left limbs since she had no control of the right side of her body. Some other folks came out of their room to see about the commotion and decided to join in. Others saw the group work and decided they wanted no part of the actual physical activity, but envied the social togetherness. Most of them counted loudly and as they did, other residents and staff took notice. This became a daily thing and something that everyone looked forward to. I was at my med-cart each day watching and encouraging everyone. I was counting the reps out loud while I also counted the doses of medications for each resident. Even Arnie the one-on-one monitor for Leslie would do some of the exercises. He could tell that some folks needed encouragement and if Arnie the Marine was sitting there doing these exercises, that meant it was probably good for the residents too.

At dinner time everyone would go back to their rooms to eat. Once dinner was over, only a few residents would return to hang out and talk, but for the most part the hot corner cooled down after supper. Most residents were not night owls and could fall asleep at any point in the day so they were usually sleeping by 1900 if they had it their way.

The next day I arrived to see Luna, Arnie the marine, and six or seven residents sitting at the hot corner. It seemed like they were resting in-between sets. I took the silence and opportunity to do one of my favorite bits. I would also test their memories and see if they remembered the bit from weeks before...

I opened my eyes real big and put on my best shocked and surprised face while smiling, "Oh. My. God!" I walked slowly towards the crowd of wheelchairs, "Is this a surprise party?! How did you guys know?!" I kept speaking very loudly while hopping and dancing around. Everyone was very confused and said nothing except Tabatha.

"What... are... you... talking... about?" She was looking around at the others and back to me almost disgusted.

"Oh," I said glumly while lowering my head, "Never mind. I thought this was my surprise party." I walked behind my desk and sat down. Arnie and Luna laughed at my joke and so did Tabatha and Lucie—it went over a couple of heads but it was still clever in my mind. Tabatha enjoyed raining on any and every parade and she told me indelicately that it wasn't a surprise and then said proudly that they were doing exercises. None of them remembered the last time I did this or at least didn't call me on my re-using of material. It was always new to them, but to my agile and nimble mind working at full capacity I was Bill Murray in *Groundhog Day*. I had little material but it was never-ending since their brains always forgot the jokes from the days or weeks before. I laughed it off and let them continue.

Leslie Dawson didn't participate but she liked to watch the others doing the exercises. Arnie and I tried to encourage her, but she just stared at everyone blankly. She didn't like talking in front of anyone but I could tell she liked being part of something. Even Jordan Cliff would come out of his room and watch everyone do their exercises. He was another one who was too tough or too proud to be caught doing exercises but he too enjoyed the company and camaraderie. At the end of each set, everyone would clap and "Woo-hoo!" Luna had found her niche and maybe her purpose. We talked at the end of the night and I told her how so many people here needed help and maybe that's why she ended up here. She rolled her eyes and didn't accept it as God's plan and I couldn't blame her. I didn't know God's plan, but I did know how to present alternative ways of looking at things and other reasons for things. I would say God works in mysterious ways, but there I would go again pretending to know of God's work.

We got a new admission to the floor sometime in late July. Her name was Rhonda Ford. She had recently suffered a stroke and was an addict/alcoholic. I had cared for her once during COVID and I remember her sneaking around in her wheelchair and tickling residents' feet at their bedside. These types of things always made me laugh, but I also remembered her being quite a terror. She was unable to communicate because of her aphasia. She would try to put words together but it just sounded like incoherent babble. She was fifty years old but the way she looked and behaved, you might mistake her for a teenager. The heroin and the alcohol most likely led to the stroke, like so many others we cared for. She wheeled around the unit and always made trouble for everyone. She continued to pet feet and took a liking to Jordan Cliff. She would hold his arm and hang on him and hug Mr. Cliff. We told her, "Hey! Rhonda, you're married! I'm going to tell your husband!" She found this very comical and would try to say something but no assembled thoughts would come out. She would cock her head to the side and stare at us with one good eye and put her index finger to her mouth, telling us to "Shhh" and keep a secret; then she would laugh. She roomed with Kylie Kennedy for about two days before Kylie demanded the supervisor move her from the room. Anything could set Rhonda off and she couldn't make her needs known, so solving the problem usually took a long time, if we ever figured it out at all. After the cup of coffee with Kylie they decided that since she was a screamer, she would fit right in with the scream queens in the corner quadruple. Donovan and Jan Konkle shared the quadruple room alone because no one could tolerate their yelling and screaming all day and night. After spending a couple of days with the real screamers, Rhonda rarely made a peep in the room anymore. I witnessed a couple of times Rhonda starting an outburst and setting off the scream queens. They yelled their obscenities at the top of their lungs. They hissed and once in a while threw things. Once Rhonda heard their rebuttal, she stopped yelling immediately.

Compared to her new roommates, Rhonda was an angelic princess and rarely misbehaved. Because her room was a certain kind of hell, she enjoyed hanging out with everyone in the hall when she could. We got Rhonda out of the room most days so she could socialize. Eventually, we figured out that, like most everyone else, music held a special place in her heart. She could be in the worst mood ever and then once you turned on some Motown music she would smile and start to sing. She'd hold up her one working hand and start swinging it around and moving her head and neck a little. Everyone thought it was adorable and even joined in most of the time.

She was like the little sister or niece of all the elderly on the floor and everyone looked after her. Despite her angry outbursts, the other residents learned to tolerate her and even pity her. The other residents combed her hair and helped feed her. They would help her drink her thickened water and point her in the right direction if she got lost down the hall. If she was misbehaving in someone's room, they would call the nurse to get her out of there. Jordan Cliff loved it when she would wheel up next to him and hold his arm and pet him. We all took to calling Jordan Cliff, "Uncle Jordan" when she was loving on him.

It was particularly heartbreaking when a younger person would suffer a stroke and their whole life was upended. I always wondered where and when the exact moment of acceptance took place—if it ever did. I was grateful when I saw cases like hers. It made me happy I got sober. The chances of stroke or wet brain significantly decreased once I stopped drinking all day, every day. Most of the residents who suffered a stroke secondary to alcohol or drug abuse had no family at all. I had to presume that their behavior and lifestyle had isolated them from their family members before their physical problems had begun. Maybe, because of their addiction, their family members abandoned them and wanted nothing to do with them. They were written off and their addiction continued to progress until eventually their addiction caused a life-changing stroke. Once the stroke would happen, and the trauma came with it, they would find themselves in a nursing home with no family or friends to visit or support them. It was truly depressing.

In my Alcohol Support Groups, we had another phrase we quoted frequently—*Jails, Institutions, or Death*. If we kept on in our habit we would end up in prison, in a psych facility, or dead. Until I started working in the nursing home and seeing all the cases related to substance abuse, I'd never considered a nursing home as an institution where an alcoholic or addict might find themselves. I felt obligated to share these stories in my Alcohol Support Groups in hopes that it might open some eyes and keep someone sober for just one more day.

Eventually, Arnie left us. Apparently, administration had forgotten that he was on the payroll through the temp agency, and he'd stayed a month or two extra. His leaving was so abrupt, that we didn't get to plan a party or even get him a card. It was sad to know he wouldn't be coming back. Leslie, due to her dementia, didn't remember him day to day, but he made friends with a lot of other residents who he helped and talked with. Arnie and I would make up stories about traveling youth choruses in North Dakota and how we'd both been in Middle Earth during the battle of The Two Towers. I would tell all the residents how I was psychic and he would correct me and say I was psycho. I would tell Tabatha and Lucie how Arnie and I were undercover narcotics agents in Brooklyn and how we took down the Zamboni crime family and how they were ice cold. I told our audience how we were badass, and Arnie would chime in and say that we weren't badasses, but bad apples and how we shouldn't be working with the elderly. Our banter and wit were constantly going on for all to watch and hear. Some listened in amazement and others just disregarded our farces. This was a source of entertainment for us as well as the residents. Luna enjoyed the stories as well even though she knew they were complete fiction. Luna and Arnie were the only ones that I could have a meaningful conversation with, and now Arnie was gone. Most of the CNAs and nurses spoke English as their second language so conversation was impossible with them, and the residents were always confused or unable to express their thoughts or ideas.

Once Arnie left, Luna took over the 1:1 monitoring post. I told her we would need her resume and a drug test for her to be officially employed by our facility. We laughed. She also became my assistant. She would sit at the hot corner for most of my shift, watching Leslie and convincing her not to walk on her own. Every time Leslie tried to get up, Luna was there to say, "Leslie! Don't get up! I'll get the nurse!" Leslie would forget Luna was there and look up, shocked to see her outside the door. She would usually lie back down after the strong direction. Because of COVID and limited human interaction, there were periods of time when Leslie didn't get up for days, sometimes even weeks. Since her muscles were contracting and her blood pooling, she couldn't walk a single step anymore, but still tried. If she managed to lift herself off the bed she would go down almost automatically, but I entrusted this task to Luna, knowing she was of sound mind and would let me know when Leslie was ready to take the walk of faith. A couple of times she would yell and I would start my wind sprint down the forty-yard hallway. When I arrived near her room I would have to decelerate to a slow walk, so I wouldn't startle her into falling as I entered her room. If I ran into any room too fast I would no doubt scare someone into a heart attack. I would try to have her sit in the bed or wheelchair. Her mind was set on doing or saying something, but when she went to express that notion, she would lose her train of thought and forget what she needed or why she'd decided to try the walk of faith.

I talked to Anita every day because she sat at the hot corner more than anyone else. Her male suitors would come and sit with her for a little while. After one suitor sat and chatted for twenty minutes, he would leave, only to be replaced by another person seeking her company. Everyone liked Anita because she would say funny things in English and they would all have a laugh. I continued to try and speak my Spanish but she responded to everything I said with her signature *"COMO?!"* It was frustrating and I found myself doubting my bilingual skills, but knew it wasn't my Spanish that was the problem. Anita was the only Spanish-speaking person I'd ever met who didn't speak Spanish. I thought her dementia might be the reason for this but then heard her speak in English after being frustrated that someone couldn't understand her Spanish. Then I heard her remembering my name from weeks before. She would also remember her medication. I thought maybe it was all an act. She could recall things from months before and bring up things that others forgot. Maybe she was just hard of hearing…

Luna and I also considered the possibility of Anita being a psychic. Somehow she knew that my parents and grandfather lived together in a town forty minutes south—she named the town and asked how all three were doing. I was completely taken aback and equally perplexed. It was most likely a coincidence, but even Luna said that Anita told her things that she had no way of knowing. She told Luna things about her mother who'd passed away years before, and other mysterious things. We marveled at the possibility that she had otherworldly connections. Anita had the potential for major blowouts with other residents. This was due to the fact that she liked to go through people's clothes when they were out of their room. She also tried to claim other people's TVs, appliances, and gadgets. When she got into these moods and focused on a particular item, we sometimes would give in and give her whatever she wanted just to appease her—as long as the other resident wouldn't miss the object. It wasn't right, but we had to keep the peace and keep Anita happy. Her bullet-proof bifocals and unkempt appearance kept everyone from suspecting her of any evil deeds. Many other residents and even staff members underestimated her ability to move around, communicate, and understand the goings-on of the unit. She was another fan favorite, even if she was forever mischievous and deceitful.

The days went on and more travelers were leaving but we still had a good core of kick-ass workers. I learned that only the very best travelers were invited back for the three-month contract extension. The more travelers that left, the less care the residents were getting. Fewer travelers meant the food trays were being handed out at a painfully slow pace. I remembered this being a problem in my first week and decided we were going to start yelling "TRAYS UP!" when the food carts arrived. They did this in the jail where I'd stayed for two months and I later learned that it was also common practice in the military. That same night I started yelling it at dinner time. Jeoffrey Pratt said, "Well they only say that in two places—in prison and in the military—and I don't see any stripes on your shoulder, soldier!" he winked and we laughed loudly. I'd told him about my alcoholic history a couple of months earlier and he probably remembered that I'd been to jail, and this didn't bother me. He continued to help everyone out on the floor, including the CNAs.

Shawna was able to get NPs and MDs to write orders for medications and other things the residents needed. She could adeptly present her case to any ordering practitioner and they would order whatever Shawna wanted. The nurse was still, and would always be, the backbone, heartbeat, and brain of the healthcare industry.

One of the orders she got was to discontinue Luna's three-times-a-day heparin. For a resident who was in bed and not moving, heparin was a necessary medication to prevent blood clots and stroke. For a couple of weeks, Luna had been getting out of bed every day, traveling the halls in her wheelchair, and conducting her daily exercise class. Shawna told the doctors this and they agreed she could come off of it. I believe that in modern medicine we prescribe way too many medications at the drop of a hat. Luna's stomach was covered in black, blue, yellow, and green bruising from the heparin. Her stomach eventually started to heal and the minute skin tears and bruises from the hundreds of injections began to clear up. On top of the improved skin integrity, she also needed three fewer injections a day and since no one likes needles, this made her very happy.

This type of thing Shawna was doing was something I would never have thought to initiate. Once I saw how she influenced the doctor's decision to discontinue the heparin I started to pay attention to what other things I could get ordered or discontinued for my residents. Up until Shawna's medication maneuver, I didn't really think nurses could do this. If I say it out loud it sounds so funny: "Call the doctor and tell them to do this!" *How silly!*

By the end of August, residents were allowed to start getting food delivered, and Luna had friends who brought her groceries weekly. They would also get her fast food and sandwiches from local sub shops. Since Luna didn't have an appetite, she rarely ate. She would distribute potato chips and crackers and other food all over the units to people who were able to have solid foods. She always checked with the nurse before giving a new resident food. In addition to her snack train, she would sing songs to some residents who never got out of bed, and tried to give company to residents who would have her. She had found her purpose and was thriving.

I told Luna to keep working out and keep losing weight. I told her Shawna and I were doing the same. We had weights in the hotel room and were also doing some bodyweight exercises. I figured talking about fitness and providing social support would continue to encourage her to keep up the exercise.

During the month of August, Shawna and I drove over an hour to go to Bellmawr's Atilis gym. They made national news when they defied the Stay and Shelter order imposed by governor Murphy. Every day they stayed open, they were fined $15,000 dollars for disobeying the law. We wanted a real pump and decided it was worth it to travel and support their cause. They had a similar mindset to ours—this shutdown was doing far more damage than the actual virus. The two owners who appeared on FOX News happened to be in the gym while we were there. We paid the day pass for the two of us and spoke to one of them, saying, "We support what you guys are doing down here. Takes a whole lot of balls." I wasn't sure what I was saying. They were basically temporary celebrities. I gave him an extra twenty dollars. "Here's for your legal defense, bud. Keep it up!"

He thanked us and told us to enjoy our workout. We stayed close to four hours in the crowded and steamy gym. Once most of the customers got past the doors they took off their face masks. Shawna and I concluded that it was definitely not safe and they definitely were not following the COVID protocols. We were guilty as well and took off our masks once we started working out. We hit every muscle group during the longest workout of our lives. It would be the only workout we would have in months and we weren't sure when we would work out again! We wanted to make sure every body part was sore for a week. It was a costly trip but well worth it for the pump.

I got floated all around the facility during this time. For every five-day work week, one of those shifts would be on another unit. I was on the 3A locked dementia unit for a shift. During the height of our facility's pandemic, the whole unit became a quarantine unit. I worked a shift or two when fourteen out of the sixteen residents had COVID at the same time, and the two who didn't have it stayed in the unit. I'm not sure why the uninfected stayed, but I deduced that management suspected the two left out of the virus' war path might be contagious after living through all the exposure to the rest of the positive cases. I can't recall if the two non-COVID cases ever got it because I didn't return frequently enough.

When I returned in August I found that two residents in the locked unit had perished from COVID, but all the others returned to their regular health and lives. The total for our facility was somewhere in the high twenties (we would have to subtract a couple of deaths because some of the residents would be passing away anyway, at a rate of about 1 or 2 per month). The residents on this floor were completely demented. Their minds were completely gone. On top of that, residents ended up on this unit because they continued to wander and always tried to elope and escape the grasps of the facility. We would find them at the corner store or walking down the street. Once they got to this floor they would never leave it. The staff held the keys to the locked door and had to be careful when entering or exiting. Many of the residents refused their medications and security was being called to the max security section almost daily.

I heard of a resident named Jed Halloway and of the terrors

synonymous with his name. He was a paranoid schizophrenic with bipolar disorder. In August, I had my first interaction with him and at first he seemed well-behaved and maybe even pleasant. I pulled my cart to his room but made sure not to turn my back to him in case he tried to get physical—this was psych nursing 101 and something my mother had told me about when she was a new nurse in a psych unit. She told me to never turn my back and always make sure I had a path to the exit. I always thought that residents might give me an easier time because of my sex and size. I was six-foot and muscular. I usually wore a camouflage bandana so I was hoping my appearance would deter Mr. Halloway from doing anything funny—or physical. I tried to be strict and assertive in the hopes of slightly and safely intimidating him. I speculated how our brief encounter would go and decided to dive right in. "Hey Jed, how are you today? Feeling okay?" I asked loudly and clearly but didn't give him a chance to respond. "I'm going to get your medication ready, okay? Feel like taking your vital signs today?" I made little eye contact and pretended to inspect the room for safety.

"No vital signs! Just the medication!" He yelled in a deep snarl.

"Fair enough! I'll get it right now," I responded firmly as stepped out to my cart.

He had a ton of meds and I took my time preparing them. He had no blood pressure medications so I didn't have to worry about obtaining the current blood pressure and marked him as a refusal for vital signs. He was on anti-depressants, anti-psychotics, regular supplements, and the list went on. I gathered all ten pills in a med-cup and took a deep, optimistic breath, ready to go in. "Okay, Jed. Here's everything, bottoms up!" I continued my short, concise dialogue.

"Okay, okay, what do we have here," he asked, talking to himself in a low snarl while he took the medication cup from me. He looked at me and then to the med-cup and back to me again. I could tell something bad was about to happen, I just didn't know what. His face went from observant and curious to absolute rage. He turned as red as an apple as if he were holding his breath violently. His eyes became wide and stared at me with absolute intensity. My first instinct was *fight!* The secondary *flight* option won out and would be the better choice in this elderly setting.

As I started to feel the sweat surface on every inch of my body, he stood up from his chair, still staring at me with violent eyes, *"I don't fucking want them! Get the fuuuuck out!"* He snarled at the top of his lungs, maintaining his intense eye contact and he threw the medication cup with the pills against the wall. "Get the fuck out! Fuck you!" Growling, he didn't make a move toward me, but I noticed his fists were clenched. I walked backward out of the room, keeping an eye on him. I closed the door and listened to his rant from the hallway. I was safe and now it became curiosity and entertainment. Psych residents and their diagnoses were particularly intriguing to anyone until it got ugly and violent. He continued to mutter obscenities in his room and never tried to come out. I imagined him pacing up and back in his room but I didn't know what he was actually doing. He said things about people not knowing him, and how dare they. He talked about killing people and getting out of the facility. At one point it sounded like he was having a conversation with himself. It sounded like he was asking himself questions and then answering them. I thought about the pills on the floor and then thought that my safety was more important. I thought that in the future I wouldn't try to give him medications again. I ultimately deemed him helpless and hopeless. This was tough for me because I was here to help, but when it came to those who didn't want my help and could be potentially violent and homicidal, I had to look after my own safety and focus on those who needed and wanted my help. It was always very difficult to give up on a resident, but I had to think of all the other starfish who needed saving. If he murdered or injured me it would take time and assistance away from all the others… a slight exaggeration, but true nonetheless.

Shawna worked in the locked dementia unit frequently and during one of these shifts, she endured an assault by a larger resident whose mind was gone like the wind. He punched her in her shoulder, and when Shawna wanted to send him to the hospital, the new supervisor Desiree, with only nine months of nursing experience, decided against it. She told Shawna she needed to work on how to talk to the resident. This was called therapeutic communication. Shawna laughed in Desiree's face and told her to try.

Desiree came onto the unit and found the resident in the wheelchair all worked up. She crouched down to his eye level to talk to him. "Hi Walter! How are you today?" Her enthusiasm could make you sick. "What happened?! Are you okay?!"

"Get the fuck out of my face," he said, and slapped her in the face.

She was athletic enough to roll with the slap and only take about thirty percent of the blow. She was embarrassed and wouldn't abandon her post.

"Now Wally, that wasn't nice. What's bothering you?!" She did a duck walk backward as she braced for more impact. Wally clenched his large fist. He must have been a mason or a lumberjack because his arms and hands were large and calloused. He cocked back his fist to his ear and was ready to strike. Desiree stood up and walked away past a smiling Shawna.

"I don't think we have to send him out, we just need to let him calm down," she said, embarrassed, as she walked off the unit.

Therapeutic communication worked well if the subject had no cognitive impairment and was open to such communication. This was never the case though—especially with demented psych residents locked in one place. Sometimes drugs and restraints were the only way to keep staff and other residents safe. Even then, doctors were hesitant to prescribe them.

It was a funny scene to see Desiree with her nine months of nursing try to enlighten a hardened and seasoned nurse like Shawna. She did this with all the other travelers—but damn it, Desiree sure did try!

During the end of summer, more and more liberties were granted to the population and with them, everyone started talking about "The second wave." I got tired of hearing that term after working five months on the front line and wanted to scream for them to *shut the fuck up*! like an agitated psych resident. I didn't think it was possible, if everyone had already gotten COVID and had built up antibodies and immunity. On top of that, we were all sanitizing our hands every six minutes, wearing masks, and social distancing. How could a second wave be possible?! Needless to say, the second wave came, but for my facility, it was in two parts. The first part was in September.

Chapter 18

September

Don't want to be...all by myself... - Eric Carmen

Starting September First, after a COVID-free August, we had one new case and so it began. Upon hearing the news, everyone rolled their eyes and huffed and puffed and waited with anxiety. No one wanted to go through another three-plus months of isolation and imprisonment. Hadn't it been enough?! And who was spreading the virus, damnit!? We still had the check-in staff at the lobby taking temperatures and *asking* us questions about symptoms and travel. As for the PPE, we only had to wear our n95s and surgical masks. I checked in through the desk, got my n95 and went to the nursing office to confirm my assignment.

The young and green Desiree pulled me into the side office and told me I would be designated COVID nurse on 1B. I wasn't too pleased, but didn't let it show. I tried to find the positives in the situation. I wondered what God had in store for me and what was the reason I was going back down to a quarantine roulette situation that I wish I could forget. Desiree told me that I would be down there for the foreseeable future and I should get used to it.

She told me how there was only one resident at the moment—well, I could get behind that! It was Alice Zimmerman and she was pleasant as a peach and had no cognitive impairment. She knew which meds she would take and when to take them. Alice was the one who argued with the traveler CNA about changing her too early, not knowing that the CNA would change her as many times as she liked. Since there was only one resident in quarantine, there was only one nurse and no CNA. The nurse was responsible for everything, including washing the resident and changing the resident's briefs. The only issue with this was that Alice refused male care. I did my best to try and convince Alice, but she was adamant about only females caring for her when it came to washing her and her private parts. So instead of stationing a CNA alongside me for the whole shift, they would pull a CNA in when she needed to be changed. The CNA would have to don full PPE at the entrance of the unit and doff the PPE when she left, and we would hope that she wouldn't spread COVID to the other unit she was returning to.

Housekeepers would walk through quarantine and I would yell at them. One of them said that it was okay to walk through the hall because the COVID was only in the room. I wondered what kind of reasoning that was, and if his supervisor was the one giving him this misinformation. To my knowledge, at that point, no one was allowed in the unit. I called the other supervisor and told her how too many people were walking through the unit carelessly. She said that there were signs up and that was all they could do. I surrendered my argument and continued to yell at people for coming through the unit. Hadn't they learned from the last six months of torture and misery and mask-wearing and global shutdowns?!

I got back to Alice, did her double vital signs, and gave her all the medications she needed. I spent much of my time on the computer listening to podcasts and watching soccer. Whenever Alice called, I gowned up as fast as I could and ran right in to help her with whatever she needed. I would call the supervisor to find an aide to come change her if that's what she needed. If she needed water or snacks I would bring them to her immediately. I felt bad for Alice because she was absolutely asymptomatic, but still tested positive. By this time we were getting weekly rapid swab tests. One of my doctor friends at the facility was telling me how the PCR test could trigger a false positive because of remnants of the virus being present. I wondered if that's what was happening here. Alice was one of the last in the facility to contract the virus during the first round of COVID. She had it in late July into early August, so I presumed her antibodies were fresh and effective. Alice was a good sport about the whole thing and she usually stayed in bed anyway so the quarantine didn't really affect her.

During her two-week stay her husband and dog came to visit her.

They could come to the window and talk on the phone. They had removed the negative pressure fans in the windows so I didn't have to worry about COVID air blowing directly onto the human-canine combo. The dog could see his mom through the window and went nuts jumping and yapping in its dad's arm. It was a cute little yorkie and it was a visit Alice desperately needed. Since she'd been living on the second floor previously, her husband would have needed a roofing ladder and some courage for a window visit. Now she was on the first floor so her husband and pup came a couple of times a week. This made me happy and did wonders for Alice's spirit and attitude.

Two days before Alice left we admitted a ninety-four-year-old half-blind and legally deaf woman to the unit. She tested positive and was in the hospital for about a week before testing negative and coming to us for "Rehab." I assumed, after staying in bed for a week while in the hospital, that it would take a toll on her walking. Not only did she normally walk, but she also did stairs! At home, before her hospital admission, she made breakfast and lunch each day and ate dinner with her grandchildren and great-grandchildren. She also did the laundry for the whole house. One week in bed would seriously complicate and degenerate her body, and getting her back on her feet was imperative. She was absolutely livid that she didn't go right home from the hospital and she constantly let us know it!

She had zero medications prescribed! Aside from the fifty percent blindness and serious hearing problems, she was otherwise healthy. I group texted my family and some friends and told them of this true champion I had the pleasure of looking after. All I had to do was take her vitals and set up her meal for her. I would also change her briefs since she didn't mind who did it. In my free time, I still watched my soccer and listened to my Glorious House of Gainz podcast, but I had a new purpose here and that was to get this nonagenarian back on her feet! I checked in on her every twenty minutes. I didn't want to bother her, but she was my only subject and I wanted to take the very best care of the single resident I had. I refer to her as a patient and not resident because her stay was temporary and she was not living with us long-term—it's the right terminology to use. I asked her if she wanted to walk and she always replied with a resounding "Yes!"

For the first two days, we only walked around her room. On the third and fourth days, I took her down the hall. She had a walker and I walked behind her. She walked the entire football field hallway and back! She wanted to keep going but I wanted her to rest for a little bit and promised her we could do more walking later. If she did go down, I would have to unnecessarily expose someone else, who would have to come in and help me get her back to bed, even if she did only weigh ninety pounds. She did this exercise on top of the physical therapy she participated in every morning and early afternoon. Every day I spoke with her daughter, who was also deaf. We had to use a third-party translator. The daughter wanted her out too, as did the grandchildren.

The resident herself made it abundantly clear that she wanted out: "I want to go!" is what she said to me every single time I entered the room. I told the family to talk to the social worker and eventually they came and picked her up. She only spent six days in quarantine and I suspect she got back to cooking her breakfasts and doing the family's laundry. She had to get back to her purpose and her service to her family!

On my day off we admitted two more patients—another ninety-year-old from another facility with COVID who would make a full recovery, and another false positive (I presumed) who also didn't want to be here. The ninety-year-old was completely bedridden and couldn't walk. His brain was completely gone and he couldn't speak any words. Physically, he was fine. All his vital signs were fine and the only thing I had to worry about was his blood pressure getting out of hand. We medicated him for that, so it was never an issue. I changed him at least two times a shift and kept him out of wet diapers. Wet diapers led to UTIs and skin tears, and at his advanced age, either of these could be deadly.

I checked on him constantly. I would check him one last time around nine and then put him to bed. I took his dentures out and cleaned them and tried to brush his gums with an oral rinse solution on a green foam cleansing tool, all the while trying to make sure he wouldn't choke on the moisture I was introducing to his mouth. After cleaning him and changing his brief again, I brought a new top sheet and blanket and tucked him in. I took a step back and admired my work, wondering how come every resident couldn't look like this? What the hell were these CNAs doing? I couldn't judge—there were a million things that could prevent residents from looking as snug as a bug in a rug, as my guy did.

In my free time I spoke to all the family members I could get on the phone; after all, I only had two to three residents at a time, so I thought providing daily updates would be a good use of my time. The other resident left after less than a week and went back to whatever long-term facility he'd come from. None of the residents within our facility, except for Alice, came to the quarantine that September. We were taking previously positive COVID cases coming to us for rehab. Some time in August our rehab team was fully back, and boy did they have their work cut out for them. I guess everyone did, but after months of people not walking, physical therapists had a tall mountain to climb to get people back on their feet. The residents that came to us for rehab may have made progress, but once COVID happened, any and all rehab improvements were completely negated. Doctors would also have to reassess all their residents upon their return as if they were all new residents to their service.

Since I treated my September quarantine assignment seriously, I didn't go anywhere else in the building. Once I was on the unit I stayed on the unit until my shift was over, and then I left the building. Some other employees didn't practice this infection prevention. They would leave through the halls to go to their car or even go to other floors to visit other staff. Quotes about weakest links and bad apples ran through my head. A whole facility of hundreds of employees could practice infection control and hand washing and properly isolating and quarantining, but all it would take was one person to pick up the virus and carry it with them down the hall, infecting everyone as they went to gossip about some meaningless topic. That was me expecting the worse, with more speculative thinking that I had to rid my mind of.

I kept attending my Alcohol Support Group online ZOOM meetings. On a Wednesday night that September I joined one of my local online ZOOM meetings in full PPE. I figured my buddies would get a kick out of it, and they did. Since I worked every Wednesday since I started my career, I couldn't continue attending my home group in person, but since all meetings were suspended, I wasn't missing anything. I stayed online for about forty minutes with my local group and then had to end the meeting abruptly to run into a room to prevent a confused elderly patient from falling. I considered that my group might think I was showing off—running away from the computer's video stream to go "save a life"—but I didn't care.

Shawna and I moved in together and this didn't surprise anyone. When you know, you know. We decided that she would stay in the Northeast to be with me. Her contract with my facility ended on September fifteenth, as did Stephanie's and a dozen other CNAs and nurses. As a nurse—an experienced one—she could work anywhere. The travel contracts and the money they brought never really went anywhere but they were starting to heat up again due to the dreaded "Second Wave."

Shawna was working about sixty hours a week, raking it in at my facility, but she needed a break. She'd paid all her debts, lent money to family, and still had plenty in the bank. She would stay at home setting up our brand new 'one bedroom with loft' apartment. During September I took a three-day weekend and we flew to Texas to get the rest of her belongings and furniture. We packed them in a U-Haul and drove the twenty-four-hour drive through Texas, Oklahoma, Tennessee, Virginia, Maryland, Delaware, and Pennsylvania. I didn't tell my facility about traveling to and through "red-zone" states—I would no doubt have to quarantine for two weeks. I didn't need the time off, nor did I think the facility could spare it. Since the travelers were completely gone, we went back to being short-staffed. CNAs with sixteen to twenty-four residents. Nurses with twenty-six to thirty-eight residents. Shawna and her cats would be living in the Northeast for the first time ever.

During the second to last day of the travelers' assignments, I heard from Shawna about Mel and Kelly abandoning their posts when they heard there were only three CNAs for eighty-something residents. They refused to work with that many residents. They left the breakfast carts with all the residents' food and walked out of the building. They ended their assignment like that, leaving the building even more short-staffed with their exit. This news absolutely killed me. They were two of the best CNAs we'd had for six whole months and this is how they chose to be remembered! It absolutely blew my mind. I compared the compassion and hard work they exhibited daily for six whole months, to the selfish and cowardly act they'd committed in just one single moment. The nurses and remaining single CNA would have to pass the breakfast and lunch trays for the whole floor. As for residents sitting in their own waste—I prefer not to think about that. I correlated this act of selfishness to the many betrayals George R.R. Martin wrote about in his famous novels. It still pains me to think about it to this day. I don't know the full story and I try not to judge but it's very hard not to. I suspect that Mel followed Kelly's lead or was somehow influenced by her—he was just too damn kind and innocent. The following day he showed up for the last day of work on his contract… I'm not sure what was said to him but he was sent home and I never saw or talked to him again and I had no desire to try and get his information.

Life went on and my requirement to satisfy the sobriety program through the Board of Nursing continued. Quest Diagnostics was where I made water for the Board of Nursing to test for drugs. They had started an appointment scheduling service to make it "safer" for customers to come in for their laboratory testing. You could not book an appointment on the same day you wished to visit the Quest center. They were usually booked one week in advance. After becoming keen on this system I started to book all my appointments every day at the 11:30 a.m. time slot, two to three months in advance. During the September quarantine, I spent one evening booking all my appointments in advance on my smart phone. I would have to register each appointment as if I were a new patient. Name, date of birth, address, type of test, date of appointment, time of appointment. It was time well spent since my facility paid for my personal clerical duties. This way, whenever I was selected to take a drug test I could show up at 11:25 and be in and out in ten minutes. Their lines were usually out the door with walk-in visits who made no appointment. I would skip the line, check in, pee in a cup, and walk out. I felt guilty skipping all these people waiting outside, but the bottom line was I had to do this three times a month now and *I was a pandemic nurse, damn it!* My time was more precious than theirs anyway—*and* I was more clever than them. I scoffed at them having to get back to their couch and collect their unemployment.

The LA Fitness near us finally reopened in mid-September, and Shawna and I were first in line for memberships after having only *really* worked out once over the last six months. We started hitting the gym five times a week and quickly noticed all the strength we had lost over the last half a year. Everyone had to wear a mask inside the LA Fitness and if you didn't, you would be quickly reminded to do so. It was finally something for us, and we enjoyed the pump every day we got to go.

The 2020 election was right around the corner and on top of the monumental presidential election there were also state elections for New Jersey. Aside from all the political positions up for grabs in New Jersey, there was also a very important "question" on the docket. Governor Murphy had, in my opinion, gotten elected two years before because he'd made a campaign promise to legalize marijuana. He won the 2018 election, but failed to fully pass the bill that would allow folks to smoke marijuana recreationally. Since the bill hit a snag, he decided the voters would determine the law, just as many other states had previously done. Once I found out about the cannabis vote I customized a green tee shirt with a marijuana leaf on it and the words, "Vote YES to legalize marijuana on November 4th!" I wore it most days we went to the gym in order to spread word about the vote. I didn't smoke marijuana but I believed it was far less dangerous than alcohol. When comparing my resume of drunkenness and foolish decisions to the nights I was smoking weed and watching TV on the couch, the evidence was irrefutable. In my opinion we should go back to prohibition, but allow the masses to smoke weed whenever they wanted. Alcohol was truly poison. No one ended up in my facility because they smoked too much reefer, but many of the stroke victims were there partially or completely because of alcohol abuse. A lot of people liked my shirt and commented on it. Some people didn't know what it meant so I enlightened them and encouraged them to tell every freaking person they knew. I also believed the medicinal benefits and potential cannabis had, should be explored free of stigma and judgement. I wouldn't get involved in talking about the presidential election itself, but figured this was an important initiative on the ballot. New Jersey would also vote for a tax break for military veterans—I told everyone these were both no-brainers regardless of which candidate they wished to vote for president.

After a slow, easy and mainly uneventful September, I would return to 2B—my home!

Chapter 19

October

Who says you can't go home - Bon Jovi

I got to my unit and said hello to all the hot corner patrons doing exercises and then ran through the halls like it was the first (or last) day of school, saying hello to everyone and asking how they were doing. I got to Lucie Greer and Julie Walton's room and saw that Julie's bed was empty. My first thought was that she was moved to another floor, although that would make no sense since she'd been in that same bed in that same room for four years. I thought maybe COVID. I thought maybe she was in the hospital. I saw that all her picture frames and belongings were gone, so I expected the worst.

I asked Lucie what happened. "Oh, honey, she passed away," she said calmly and sadly.

"Oh man, do you know what happened?" I figured lack of care was what killed her ultimately. Lucie gave me a bunch of different answers, but it was clear she didn't really know. Apparently, she went to the hospital for something unrelated to COVID and never came back. I tried to believe that even if I was there for her, I probably couldn't have helped. I'm sure her decline had something to do with her not getting out of bed as often as she used to. I didn't shed any tears, but was deeply saddened. I thought because of my calloused COVID heart, my residents wouldn't get any more of my tears. I loved taking care of Julie and the way she always smiled at me. It was like she knew my secret past of alcoholism and how I rose out of my self-made flames to become the man I was today, and was proud of me for all that.

"Oh Julie loved you so much honey," Lucie said, trying to make me feel better.

How would you know, Lucie? She told you this? "Thank you, Lucie, I appreciate that." I walked out and back to the hot corner to chat with the exercise committee and tell them how proud I was of all of them. I had to focus on what I could do for the ones who were still with us.   L u n a told me how great their exercise was going despite my absence. Undeterred by my leave, Luna reported that most days they were all out there doing their sets and reps. I got a reputation as drill sergeant and fitness coach, which I was pleased with. It became a common occurrence and everyone expected them all to be there each day after lunch and before dinner. If sets and reps weren't being completed, staff would ask what was happening and where everyone was. Eventually, I bought Luna a speaker to connect to her iPad, so they could listen to music while they worked out. I told them that this was the way I worked out, and they loved it. The added benefit for me was that I could listen to the music without being an earbud-wearing *bad* nurse.

My fall risk, Leslie Dawson, could often be found with the group and if not, Luna made sure to keep an eye on her in her room, even while leading the group in their exercises. Luna was my right hand and knew who she had to watch out for, among other responsibilities she had. When I left the unit for a few minutes I would give her the Robert De Niro, "Meet the Parents" double fingers to my eyes, then to hers, then to the cart, signaling that I was leaving and she had to keep guard. She continued to thrive and I have to say she must have felt a responsibility for a lot of those residents. She was younger than most of the residents by fifteen to thirty years, but I nicknamed her Aunt Luna anyway. Some residents took the name and ran with it. Others didn't remember her name or who she was.

Anita Gregg could always be found in the circle doing her exercises. She would constantly look around to make sure others were doing it, or maybe compare her technique to others. She started calling me Macho Man. She knew that I would leave at 11 p.m. each night and would confirm my departure every shift. I continued to try speaking my Spanish to her, but she never could fully understand me. Occasionally she would speak in perfect English, leaving the staff and other residents puzzled. We decided not to try and figure anything out in terms of her cognition or linguistic abilities. She was an enigma and maybe we weren't meant to figure her out.

Every day I made sure Jim Moss could hear the classic rock playing from his bed. He was right at the entrance of the quadruple room so if Luna put the speaker towards the utility room corner, he could hear it perfectly. He still refused to get out of bed, but enjoyed listening to the music and camaraderie. The scream queens might hear it if they weren't in an active spell of yelling. My theory was that the music would calm the screamers down, but I guess we just never found the right genre.

Tabatha was miserable and let everyone know it hourly. Her favorite line was, "This...is... ridiculous!" As if once she used the "R" word, we would stop the press, stop what we were doing, and get her transferred to a five-star facility with a personal assistant for her every beck and call. She saved all her breath and emphasis for the word *ridiculous* at the end of her sentence and shouted as loud as she could every day. Apparently, her granddaughter passed away over the summer so I tried to practice extra patience with her, and especially all her complaints. Her granddaughter had been only thirty years old so it was an absolute tragedy. I told her how sorry I was to hear the news and that I would pray for her and her family—and I did. Tabatha wanted to be mask-free, she wanted to go to activities, and she wanted to eat in the dining room. She especially wanted to see her family who were still not allowed to visit. I had to put our feud aside for that time and take extra special care of her.

Since mid-September saw all the travelers depart, the resident count per nurse and CNA doubled overnight. Because of the decreased amount of help, residents suffered even though we weren't really going through COVID war time. Leslie Dawson rarely ever tried to walk or get out of bed on her own. I suspected that her brain understood her weakened legs just couldn't handle it anymore.

After Corey's two-week stint in quarantine and not getting out of bed a single time, such was the case with him. I weighed the quarantine and isolation and risk of death versus the direct and indirect consequences the world would face as a result of it, and whether it was worth shutting everything and everyone down. I decided the world suffered greater from being shut down than civilization losing a couple million citizens. I then thought of the overtaxed hospitals and ERs who had to deal with the patients whose bodies were riddled with the virus. Even if the survival rate was so high, the hospitals still got the sickest people no matter what. Because of this I decided a lockdown was absolutely necessary. We as a country were not well behaved—we were addicted, overweight and generally non-compliant with any type of medicine or healthy habits. We were doomed to begin with. I recall within the first week or two of quarantine seeing that family have a barbecue in their front yard on a warm March day. There were at least ten people and only half were wearing masks and none social distancing. I thought they were being selfish and stupid. It was like hitting your head with a sledgehammer if you had a migraine in hopes it would ease the pain.

Another case of absolute decline was Brenda Keller. I met her in the early summer on the third floor, where I was seldom stationed. She was confused and only oriented to herself. She didn't know where or when she was. Physically she sat in her wheelchair and was still able to wheel up and down the long hallways all day long, talk to staff, listen, and respond to simple commands. She would talk constantly, but her sentences rarely made sense. She would also laugh a loud and hearty high-pitched laugh— sometimes at nothing or at inappropriate times. She arrived on 2B that October and was Lucie Greer's new roommate. Lucie was a grandmother-type and welcomed her new roommate, looking after her without me having to ask.

Brenda was still in her wheelchair wheeling around, just a little less than usual. She was generally pleasant but sometimes out of nowhere, she would lock eyes with me as I attempted to provide care or administer medication and say "Fuck you! You're a bitch!" It was completely out of character for her otherwise pleasant personality. It was as if she was possessed by a demon during a two-second time span. The evil spirit would be gone as fast as it came and she would turn back to her normal, jovial self. If I took these outbursts personally I would be an absolute fool. She would come to the hall and I would tell her to watch my six, and she would wheel next to me and my cart. It was funny because I can't recall ever having to explain to her what 'watching my six' meant. She would hear the order and wheel to wherever I was. Brenda was on my right and Luna on my left.

Staff members joked that I was starting a gang—I countered and called it the friendship circle and that anyone was welcome.

Brenda couldn't follow along with the exercises too well. She tried sometimes but would lose focus after a couple of reps. Luna would sing childhood nursery songs to her when Brenda seemed troubled or looked uneasy. Brenda didn't sing along but got quiet and listened when Luna started to sing. She would fall into a deep stare while looking at Luna. We couldn't tell if she enjoyed the songs, but she was definitely entranced in some kind of way. Whatever trouble Brenda was having, it melted away while she was serenaded by Luna's "You are my sunshine." This song would go a long way in my facility.

I enjoyed my October the best I could. The halls were quieter since the departure of our traveling angels, but the rooms grew louder with the shouts at the presidential debates and everything else going on. Residents missed Mel and Bridget and Kelly and asked where they were, every day. They asked for Shawna and Stephanie and hoped that maybe they would return some day. If they did return it would be for bad reasons, so I hoped we wouldn't see them again. Although Shawna and I moved in together after four months of dating, I didn't really feel comfortable letting my residents know about our situation—not that we were doing anything wrong or anything. I guess my ego was worried what residents like Lucie would think, knowing I'd been in a relationship when I'd first started at the facility.

Luna knew of our blossoming romance because she had no cognitive impairment, and I knew she could keep a secret. Shawna had also asked Luna about me, so she'd known Shawna had been interested.

During October we had a COVID scare which sent everyone into quarantine. We all griped and rolled our eyes. We had suffered enough and no one wanted to be confined to their rooms ever again—we'd had enough for a lifetime. After a couple of days, the resident was retested and showed a negative result, so we were able to continue our new normal life. Masks on everyone, everywhere we went. No one was pleased with the new apparel but it beat sitting in their rooms all day, every day.

Jared Bartell was still roaming the halls looking for cookies and confrontations. Josh Lemon gave him the latter. Earlier in the year, it was reported that Jared had struck Josh in the chest with a closed fist. Since then I was on the watch to prevent any more violence. I'm not sure what the administrators did to remedy this situation because the two constantly got into the food cart whenever the meals were dished out. One particular day, Jared was intimidating Josh and actually grabbed the front wheels of his chair, trying to tip him backward.

I ran over and yelled at the top of my lungs, "Jared! Stop!"

He backed away and I wheeled Josh to the other side of the facility. I talked—actually yelled at the Director of Nursing regarding the incident. At the end of the one-sided conversation, I told her I would call the police the next time I saw Jared get violent. I had a feeling that Jared thought he was immune to the justice system because he was a resident in a nursing home. The Director of Nursing didn't object, but rather agreed with my plan of action.

I ran back upstairs where the supervisor was talking to Jared and told them both I would be calling the police the next time he committed violent acts. Jared responded in kind with threats of beating my cracker, white boy ass. I then yelled the line I'd rehearsed so many times in my head on the way back up to the unit for the conversation that actually happened, "They have insulin in jail, Jared!" I figured I got him good. I thought I might get in trouble for what I said, but the seasoned supervisor said nothing regarding my choice of words.

I thought about the confrontation later that night and concluded that that was the loudest screaming match I had been in since I got sober. Even in the diner, fighting with able-bodied chefs, I never got that loud. Since then, Jared was better behaved and I like to think that it's because he now understood that all jails and prisons had nurses to administer medications. Maybe he got the point!

Jared and I ignored each other as best we could. We would sometimes have to avoid each other in the hallways when passing each other. Residents and staff would continue to yell "TRAYS UP!" at every meal, and this infuriated Jared. I got a strange satisfaction from this when I saw the steam coming out of his ears each mealtime. I figured the shouts might disturb other residents too, but I figured the prompt delivery of hot food outweighed the uncomfortable moment a few residents had when everyone was yelling about the food's arrival.

The "Second Wave" chatter continued and dominated a lot of

conversation. We collectively held our breath and hoped a vaccine would appear miraculously before it occurred, and our lives would return to normal. The vaccine was the only bit of hope we held on to. We heard of trials going well and possibly a December date for health care workers and the elderly living in nursing homes. The nursing homes continued to garner attention from the press. The press loved spewing the toxic statistical sludge for the nation to hear and fear. I wondered how it made the residents feel since they were basically the center of attention for these stories. I held on to the hope that the second wave had already hit, and since September had come and gone, we wouldn't have quarantine COVID units anymore. Boy, wrong again!

Chapter 20

November

Out of all the characteristics and traits a great nurse must have that I mentioned previously, I forgot the most important one! An iron stomach! The successful nurse can have all those traits, but needs an iron stomach to truly excel!

Going into November, the list of holidays and family events that had been canceled or I'd missed, kept growing. I missed our annual Greek Easter, our annual family picnic, July fourth, and my cousin's wedding. I couldn't go to the wedding because I'd been stationed on COVID quarantine all of September and their wedding had been right in the middle of the month. I would now spend all of November in quarantine and miss an outdoor Thanksgiving my family was hosting. I had probably built up antibodies from my suspected case that were still functional, but the risk of spreading it to my virus-free family members, who'd been on complete lockdown, was too great. By this point, I decided that if and when a vaccine came out I would have to be the first one in line, just so everyone would shut the fuck up and we could get back to a semi-normal life. My siblings and parents would feel better about me visiting if I were vaccinated since I worked on the front lines of a nursing home. I didn't want to get my nieces or nephews sick, nor my parents or grandfather.

Shawna took a travel contract starting in mid-November and went to California for work. She was stationed in California working at a COVID nursing home herself. The virus was running rampant on the west coast and Shawna was right in the middle of it. Everything was shut down and she reported ghost towns all around her San Jose area. She did a six-week assignment and would spend Christmas and New Years at a Chinese family's Airbnb. I stayed home in Jersey and took care of her cats, Keena and Moki. I did the best I could with them and they kept me company every night I got home to the large, empty apartment. I had never owned cats and considered myself a dog person, but Moki, the siamese cat, took a liking to me and would sit on my lap as I watched sports and other TV series. Keena, the handicapped kitty was still unsure of who I was and what I was doing. She showed me no affection, never let me pet her, but always accepted the food I would give her each day and night. Shawna and I texted every day and talked on the phone almost every night. I told her how her cats were and if they'd done anything funny that day. I would also tell her if they were pooping regularly, or if they had vomited. It was like I was giving a feline nurse-to-nurse report each night. She would tell me of the interesting characters in California and what her residents were like. She and I were dealing with the same resident population, who had the same problems, but on opposite coasts. Limited staffing, COVID scares, and oxygen desaturation were our topics of conversation. She would be back in early January to check on me and the cats and find another place to go to. Everyone still had to get the COVID money while it was around; they had to strike while that figurative iron was hot because it wouldn't last forever!

On my days off I would meander around the house and watch European soccer. They were back to it and playing their seasons. I watched UEFA Champions League and all the other top leagues if there were Americans playing in them. I had all the streaming apps for all the different leagues to watch our young Americans abroad. No fans were allowed in the stadiums and I found that the pandemic was always surrounding and consuming me. It was more depressing scenes and sights, but at least we finally had our soccer!

On election day I remember I had the day off and I watched the coverage from my laptop since I didn't like paying too much money for cable. The enormity of the presidential race had me glued to my computer, watching the red state/blue state maps and their percentages. I watched the coverage with the same fervor and excitement I would a Champions League soccer game. It was exciting and surely entertaining, but I prayed that whoever won would lead the country in the right direction and we as a nation would begin to heal. I prayed that there would be no riots or fighting over the results. I learned that night that the marijuana vote had passed, it would soon be legal for New Jersey residents to smoke pot legally, and was very happy for everyone who smoked weed. The veterans also got their property tax breaks!

I went to bed indifferent about the pending presidential election results—I couldn't control the outcome and wouldn't waste any more time on it. Regardless of who won I would still be in my PPE, on my COVID unit in my own corner of the world.

The whole month of November at my facility was absolutely insane. I was designated COVID nurse again and the admissions kept coming. Thanks to our Director of Nursing and our facility's monster healthcare network, we became the designated COVID facility for our region of New Jersey. We would take the positive cases from all our sister facilities in our area, as well as new rehab COVID cases, in addition to our own residents who were testing positive. I started November with five patients on the floor; one patient was our resident from the third floor. The other four were a combination of new rehab admissions and residents from our affiliated facilities. My first night I admitted another patient, bringing our new total to six residents.

It was me and another CNA for the first two weeks as our resident count quickly reached eighteen. I had to take double sets of vitals on everyone and pass their medications at 1700 and 2100. I had no free time for breaks and usually left well after midnight each night. I kept getting new admissions daily, and two in one night became a common occurrence. They were generally messy and time-consuming. For an admission you had to page the admitting doctor and confirm the resident's medications, one by one. The doctor would either confirm, or discontinue the medications. The doctor would also order labs, ultrasounds, chest X-rays, EKGs, and tons of other stuff—even if the resident had just had these tests done the night before at another facility. We had to hand-write the medication in our Medication Administration Record as well as on a physician order sheet. We then had to fax the physician order sheets individually to two separate pharmacies. We then had to complete a head-to-toe assessment on each resident. We had to check their neurological status, auscultate their lungs, inspect their bowels, assess their genitals, and check every inch of their skin for any pressure wounds or skin tears. After all this, we would have to document our findings... in ink... in a sixteen-page packet. We then had to complete a fall risk evaluation, a bed rail evaluation, and a skin tear assessment, and I'm sure I'm missing another couple of assessments.

We then had to complete care plans for each individual resident and what their exact needs were. For a care plan, we had to choose all the nursing diagnoses that applied, the interventions we could implement, and the goals for each of the diagnoses. The stack of papers we had to complete was as thick as a bible, and it seemed like every other day I was doing two of them!

Some nights I didn't leave until 2 or 3 a.m. On a good night, a night nurse would come in early to help me, or a supervisor would come and do the medications for me. Some paperwork I left incomplete, knowing that it might come back to me. I could play dumb and pretend I didn't know it was part of the admission paperwork. I could say it wasn't in the pre-made packet I received which was a half-assed excuse, but I was exhausted each day and found myself taking a lot of shortcuts. I did all the important paperwork and focused on the medications and the new orders the MD wanted. A lot of people were tired and burnt out and I anticipated that no one would be double-checking every single page of my admission paperwork—they wouldn't even want to enter the COVID unit to do so! At this point in my young nursing career I was no stranger to being tired and burnt out, so I started to do the bare minimum when it came to paperwork. Most of the patients would be leaving after their two-week stay, and their paperwork would become useless once they got back to their home facility anyway.

We had one patient from another facility who was thirty-four. He had diabetes, a history of seizures, and Marfan syndrome. He showed no signs or symptoms of the COVID and his breathing was almost perfect. He knew how to care for himself. He knew all about his medicines and how to treat his diabetes. He had been living at another facility for a couple of months for rehab. We didn't exactly hit it off, but I wanted to ensure a full recovery for him so I was extra kind to him. He was only a couple of years older than me, and I wanted him to live a long life to the best of his ability. I had to do my best for the fraction of his life that he relied on me. I constantly checked on him and let him know I cared. He always said thank you, but was always in a neutral mood and I couldn't judge him for it.

I found out that he loved underground rap and was also a moderator for a mental health chatroom/organization online. I could get behind that, and I commended him for his work. Mental health was everything and it was getting more and more attention as time went on. Talking to someone about your emotional and mental problems was important to living a healthy life. Luckily for me, I got to share openly whenever I wanted, with my ever-growing network from my Alcohol Support Groups. I wanted the world to experience what I had with my new friends and family from my Alcohol Support Groups. I was glad to see there were other people realizing that social support and mental health were a vital part of living a happy life. The patient got an early COVID negative test and was out of there in about eight days. I was happy for him and wished him luck and told him to keep up the mental health support.

Another youngster we got was forty-three years old. She'd suffered a stroke a month before and came to us from the hospital. Her name was Thuy and she was Vietnamese. She had a fun accent and despite the bad luck she was dealt, she had a great attitude and was always so very grateful. You could bring her a four-ounce cup of water with no ice or straw and she would scream, "Thank you! Thank you! Thank you, my friend!" Caring for residents like her reenergized nurses and gave them a sense of gratitude. When you came across a resident like Thuy who couldn't use one half of her body and could barely speak coherent sentences, you started to realize the blessings you had and what you should be grateful for. She made me feel appreciated and that went a very long way when most of the other residents were cranky, foul, and sometimes just plain rotten. Thuy roomed with an older lady, Vicky, who never stopped screaming. Despite the chaos her roommate constantly incited, this didn't bother Thuy. Thuy must have possessed some sort of inner tranquillity or zen—or maybe just some good headphones.

Vicky was a resident who would scream at anything and anyone. She refused to take any of her meds and was rarely quiet. Occasionally she would play with her excrement, but never went as far as to throw it. I called the previous facility she came from and they said this was not her baseline behavior. I wondered if COVID was now affecting her brain and its processes. I had noticed similar behavior from at least two other residents who normally had a calm demeanor and rarely made trouble. It had to have been COVID making these residents mad. We did the best we could with Vicky, but at some point, the staff had to weigh their own safety versus the needs of the resident. If she absolutely had to be changed, we would forcefully and administer care, hoping that she would comply, and we wouldn't be covered in feces by the end of the escapade. Other things we would let lie out of fear of injury to her and us. We certainly didn't get paid enough to be getting assaulted constantly.

One of the other residents who constantly misbehaved and yelled was Vince Kellogg. He had no prior history of combative and violent behavior, but certainly fit the bill during his stay. He refused medication and constantly asked for soda. I got him a soda one time hoping to bribe him into taking his blood pressure medication and letting us take his blood sugar, but he still didn't let us do anything—I felt like a fool who got conned by a smelly, toothless charlatan. The family and I considered the change in setting may have been the reason for his erratic and aggressive behavior, but too many COVID cases this time around had similarities of insane behavior to be sure.

After about ten days with us, his heart stopped. Magnus, a male CNA and a friend of mine, discovered that Vince was unresponsive and wasn't breathing. Magnus yelled for me and the other nurse at shift change and we came running in. Rita and I felt for a pulse and couldn't find one. Magnus started chest compressions, Rita got on her cell phone, and I got the code cart. The code cart was missing the Ambu-bag to administer oxygen through his mouth. The most important thing was the chest compressions. We called a code overhead and several nurses came to help. The supervisor came as well. Magnus did five minutes of chest compressions before the EMS came with an Ambu-bag. I took over for about two minutes, breaking four ribs of the already deceased in the process! It was a disgusting feeling that haunted me for the next couple of hours. I didn't stop the chest compressions in hopes that a miracle or these hopeless compressions might bring him back. We carried on for what felt like fifteen minutes more. We filled the EMTs in on the story, and resident's history, and how he'd been refusing all meds and barely eating. One of the EMTs listened to our summary of non-compliance and violent behavior while continuing the chest compressions. He jokingly asked, "Well, you want us to leave him like this?"

I scoffed and said, "No, no."

Magnus blurted out, "NO! Man!"

The EMT was taken aback and must have been embarrassed because he apologized right away and said something about trying to lighten the mood. He was just making a joke, which I thought was clever but maybe inappropriate—either way, I didn't take offense to the joke and the resident remained deceased.

During that time before paramedics came with an AED, I had to admit that no one had seen him since 1430—approximately an hour before we noticed his heart had stopped. I hadn't done a round on my patients that day to make sure they were alive and safe. I was embarrassed that I hadn't had eyes on him when I came in. Whenever a nurse takes over a unit, you have to always confirm that all the residents you are responsible for are alive and well, safe, and accounted for. You want to make sure no one is dead, no one is about to fall, and no one has eloped and left the facility. This was nursing 101 and I failed at this fundamental. I felt shame and embarrassment, but certainly learned my lesson. The paramedics put the electrodes on his chest and waited for a heartbeat. Nothing was there so they started shocking him. After three rounds of shocks, they called the time of death.

I was impressed with Magnus's reaction and leadership and I commended him for it. I thanked him for doing such a great job. He wasn't too bothered by our patient's departure to the other side and I wasn't either. We had been dealing with death and depression for eight months now and had become accustomed to it. In addition to our calloused hearts and souls, the deceased was not one of our regular residents so we had no real emotional connection to him. Our relationship with this patient was one of seven days and of bitterness and frustration. If it had been someone who'd lived at our facility it probably would have been a little harder on all of us. If it was someone like Evelyn I would have taken it harshly. I would have also been the nurse on shift to let her die.

I texted my sisters and mother on the *shift report* group thread and asked if it was the medication refusals that did the resident in. I asked them if this may have been on me. I asked myself if I could have done better to get him to take his meds. There were too many other residents who wanted and needed my help to sit and bargain in a room with an unruly resident who behaved like an absolute savage. My sisters and mother collectively told me that I had no control over the medication refusals, but I should have rounded the moment I arrived on the unit. My ego came back and I was angry they said that. I knew I fucked up and didn't want to hear it from anyone else—especially my family. I felt shame and embarrassment all over again. Would it have changed anything?

I called Vince's family. I called the doctor. I called the funeral home. I apologized to the sister of the resident profusely. She was in shock but I could tell she accepted that since the diagnosis of COVID, death was a possibility. I talked to her days before and said despite not taking any medication, he was physically doing okay. I told her he was still strong and eating decently, but experiencing some psychosis here and there. She was grateful for both the phone calls I made to her. Both his sister and I were unsure of who had to make the funeral arrangements so I wound up doing so. It turned out it is always the family's responsibility.

When I got on the phone with the funeral home I made sure to tell them that it was a COVID unit—that the undertaker they were sending to pick up the body would have to wear an n95. I told the person on the phone at least three times about the COVID status pick-up. I told them if they didn't have an n95 I would meet them outside with one. Two hours later the mortician came waltzing in with just a surgical mask. I had been waiting for him, knowing it was a possibility that he might enter without the proper PPE. I stopped him at the beginning of the hall, waving my arms, shouting "Stop! Go back out!"

He wasted no time in wheeling his stretcher around and getting out the door. He went through the laundry room, through the housekeeping supply room, and back outside into the chilly autumn air.

I followed him out and opened the door behind him. "Bro this is a COVID-positive unit and the body you're getting was COVID positive. I told your dispatcher all this on the phone—did they not tell you?!" I said, out of breath, second-guessing my report to the dispatcher. But I knew I'd said those things multiple times.

"No, no one told me anything. They just gave me the name and the address." He looked embarrassed. I didn't really care about his embarrassment and just wanted him to be safe.

"Damn. I know I told the woman I spoke to when I called." I rolled my eyes a little bit. But maybe I didn't know the full story.

He pulled a duck-billed n95 from his glovebox that was dirty and half-crumpled. I told him I would find a new one for him.

I spent the next ten minutes looking for the supervisor. It was Sarita, and we spent another ten minutes looking for the boxes of n95s in our supply room. We finally found some and I took some extra for my unit. I brought the mask to the grim reaper waiting outside. Instead of scythe and hood, he had gurney and n95. We walked through the housekeeping supply room and the laundry room back through the unit. I stopped him at the entrance and grabbed him a gown. He had his own gloves. I offered him some goggles but he refused, which was a good thing because I had no eye protection to give him had he accepted my offer, and even less of an idea as to where to find some. He must have been used to this COVID business and wasn't worried about his eyes. He wasn't likely to get splash damage from a corpse, so we walked down the long hallway to the room. I offered help but he declined and I let him have his time with the body. The undertakers never needed help loading the bodies onto their stretchers. There were several 250-plus pound residents that the morticians took away singlehandedly and never needed help. I envisioned them chanting some Latin and levitating the body from the bed to the gurney. He took the body, thanked me for my preparedness, and was on his way. I watched him wheel down the hall and around the corner out of view. I sat down and breathed and tried to gather myself. As I was sitting, the imaginary game show host with his long thin microphone came to mind and I pictured him saying in a solemn tone, "*Thanks for playing Covid Roulette.*"

I sat down and breathed for a little bit. We had two nurses and two CNAs for our twenty-eight residents. This type of event could have ruined someone's day, but I thanked God for the way it ended. Despite losing a mortal soul, all the staff was safe, the family was aware and we could go on to caring for others. I hoped Vince was at rest with God now and I prayed for his soul.

Through the month of November, I did the best I could with what I had. I took care of Thuy and others who would have my help. For the ones who gave me a hard time, I put forth minimal effort. I understood that their actions were a direct result of their brain being damaged from dementia and/or COVID, but it made no difference when it came to prolonged and unnecessary exposure to the virus. I felt terrible about these certain situations but if I couldn't take care of myself, I couldn't take care of others. The first thing they teach you in my Alcohol Support Groups is to get your act together and take care of yourself before you go helping others. Helping others was vital to my sobriety, but I had to be healthy myself in every way before I could render help and support to anyone else. The same principle applied here in healthcare and particularly during a pandemic.

We sent another resident to the hospital and never saw him again. His oxygen was desaturating to between 80 and 90% and I called EMS myself. I tested his oxygen on three different pulse oximeters and confirmed he was going to crash. I sent the resident out without asking the MD. I thought about what Sarita would do or say and that's what helped me decide to send him. The MD was notorious for taking hours to call back. I left the message with the answering service while the EMTs wheeled the resident out on their stretcher. He called back over an hour later. I prepared for the screaming match that would certainly ensue. I played it in my head a thousand times during the hour-plus of waiting for his return call. The doctor would say this and that, and then I would scream back, "*You never called back! What was I supposed to do?! I had to make the executive decision!*" And then it would be over and he would admit defeat and apologize. My alcoholic thinking got the better of me in this situation. An hour of stewing in this conversation that never happened, and within a minute it was over and rather pleasant. He asked who gave the order and I said, "We decided we had to send him because of his oxygen saturation. We couldn't keep it up with the non-rebreather."

"Probably needs a ventilator. You did the right thing. Thanks. Have a good night."

And with that, we hung up. I was flustered and rattled and frazzled waiting for the release from the telephone screaming match confrontation that never came. I figured he was probably at home sipping a whiskey neat, eating a steak, listening to smooth jazz, cool as a cucumber. I felt silly about how ramped up I got and laughed in my head. I then began to process the conversation and saw how the doctor had agreed with my decision and thanked me for it. Maybe at this point, I became a real nurse, assessing real life-or-death situations and making real life-or-death decisions. More roller coasters and more emotions—that was nursing for you. I decided that since the doctor didn't object to my decision to send the resident out, I would be able to write the telephone order to send the resident out. I felt like a big shot, making big decisions in big-time situations and my ego was swelling. I couldn't turn my ego off but I could certainly turn it down. I told myself to get on with it and focus on the task at hand. This whole situation could happen again in five minutes. As for the patient, we never saw him again and assumed he had passed on to the other side. He'd been kind and compliant. He'd made jokes that weren't funny and was a good sport given the circumstances. He had an uneasy air of doom and despair about him—he'd mentioned several times about dying from COVID and I'd shooed it away and tried to change the subject. I told him the same thing everyone else heard from me. "Breathe deep and just get through the day—you don't want to get pneumonia." I'd tidied up his room, called his wife for him, and did everything I could in the days leading up to his hospital admission. He'd let me help him and he'd been grateful. He was from Eastern Europe and quirky and we got along well. He was on the younger side, maybe in his sixties. He'd had the big three diagnoses—hypertension, diabetes, and COPD. He would no doubt be on a ventilator. We never called to get an update from the hospital. My reasoning was that they were too busy and maybe he had already passed. I also reasoned that if he was going to come back to us, they would call for a nurse-to-nurse report.

Besides those reasons, I just didn't have time. More admissions were rolling in as we were discharging them at the same rate, which meant tons of paperwork and coordination between all the internal staff and outside receiving facilities and families. I felt bad I couldn't follow up with him but it just wasn't realistic. All I could do was pray. I prayed for him the night the ambulance picked him up and asked God to keep him safe if that was His will.

Outside of my COVID tour of duty, I was still trying to do all the things I needed to do to maintain my sobriety and my spiritual fitness. The gyms were open but without Shawna, my workout buddy, I wasn't going to the gym. I was doing a hundred pushups and sit-ups each day instead, but I missed going to the gym. I did my Alcohol Support Groups online as well as my weekly Board of Nursing support meeting. Many of the other nurses were sick of COVID, just like me.

The only positives of COVID were that we got hazard pay for a brief time, and that family wasn't allowed to visit. We were saddened that patients and residents couldn't see their family members, but sometimes they could be too involved and overbearing. Instead of seeing them in person and asking about every little thing, we would get short weekly phone calls where we gave them an overall summary of their loved one's status. I told my Board of Nursing support group about how I was back on COVID and got their sympathy and their "Hang in there," encouragement. It was nice to know others were thinking of me and some were praying for me and my navigation through another wave of the virus. The other nurses knew exactly how I was feeling and could relate to what I was going through, and that made it a little easier. I was certain that the rest of the COVID Nurse population didn't have this support and didn't seek any either. They would let their emotions bottle up inside and marinate—and that was just not healthy. My group of sober nurses and I coped with the stress and grief the right way. I could just imagine all the other nurses self-medicating to get through these strenuous times. Talking about things that were stressing or depressing you was a healthy way to express and release those emotions. Just like Alcohol Support Groups, the social support did wonders for anyone going through extreme adversity. I wished the whole world would find their own weekly support group. By seeking help from others through social support I was able to be the best version of myself and help dozens of others because of my peak mental health.

I still did admissions almost every night, and on double admission nights, Sarita would come and help me. She would confirm certain beliefs and practices I was employing before she arrived to help me, and it made me feel smart and confident. I was doing the things a super nurse would do, as well as thinking like one too.

Sarita had been the evening supervisor for a couple of months since Desiree's departure over the summer. She was a true leader and one of the only experienced nurses we had left. She told me she was looking for another job as well and I was happy for her. What we did here in this facility was pass out pills. I hardly considered it nursing; we cared for the elderly and diseased. We hoped we could keep them comfortable as their clock ran out. The true and talented nurses belonged in hospitals and ERs, helping the younger population fight their ailments and get back to living the rest of their lives—in my opinion. I was grateful for her help and told her so every time she came. I had a feeling she liked working with me as well. Despite going to nursing school seven years before, I believed I had a good head on my shoulders, especially working with the traveling hero nurses who taught me all the important things. Sometimes Sarita would come and hang out in the COVID unit with me as if she was hiding from the rest of the building and just needed a breather. She had her n95 so she wasn't worried about COVID droplets... at all! Although Sarita never stayed for *too* long.

Towards the end of November, I remember one particular admission who brought me a second wind and new life to my COVID tour of duty. His name was Jack Kirk and I entered his room not knowing who he was. "Hello Jack, I'm your nurse, David. I'm going to ask you a ton of questions and complete your admissions paperwork. For the court's records, can you state your name and date of birth?" I quipped while smiling.

"Jack Kirk, July 3rd, 1968." He stated his name laughing.

Ah yes. Good patient. Good audience. Good customer. I can work with this. "Very good! We have confirmed your identity and your orientation to self. Do you know what time it is right now? How about today's date? Do you know where you are?" I moved around his bed, lifting his covers up, and inspecting his skin from head to toe. I made eye contact with him and knew immediately that I had met Jack somewhere before. I started to wonder when and how. Before my brain could find the answer he gave me the answers to the questions I asked.

"About 7 o'clock. November 27th, 2020. I'm in Norwich Rehab Center. I like your bracelet." He answered the questions in a monotonous tone but smiling. I was worried I'd insulted him with the silly questions—*but everyone had to answer them!*

"Oh yeah. One Day At a Time, buddy! That's the way I live my life!" It clicked that I had seen him around the meetings in the area, "You must be in the fellowship..." my mind was racing. I thought that I must know him through the fellowship of Alcohol Support Groups. I tried to place him at which meeting I might have met him. Maybe he just liked the bracelet and he just happened to be the conductor on my train or the guy at Home Depot who'd helped me pick out paint a year ago.

"Yes, I am. I used to go to meetings around here when they were in person." He was calm and cool. Alcohol Support Groups no doubt taught him his relaxed demeanor in times of trouble.   *Match calamity with serenity.*

"Ah yes. Of course. I forget where we met but it will definitely come to me." It was like a TV Crossover event and I was so excited. I finished the rest of the paperwork and the hundred questions. I told him we would take excellent care of him. I told my CNAs that Jack was a member of the church I went to. It wasn't exactly a lie because we predominantly met in church basements and side rooms and spirituality was a large part of our sobriety. Once I told a few people, I knew that I could rely on the healthcare industry's culture of gossip to spread through the building. When staff knew that a resident was connected to an employee they got extra attention and care—even if it was just a "Hey, you okay? Do you need anything?" It made the resident feel looked after and cared for.

"Alright I'll be back in a little bit with some forms and probably some more questions I missed," I chuckled as I left the room. The new energy made the end of my shift fly by. While I was doing the paperwork the memories of him came back to me and were clear. I met him at my home group on Wednesday nights at 7:30 p.m. It was a smaller meeting and he wasn't exactly a regular but I remembered him because he would always mention how he got sober in Vegas. I hopped up and walked back to his room.

"Vasilios Boulevard. Presbyterian Church. You got sober in Vegas!" I practically shouted at him with excitement.

"That's it, man! You take your bike everywhere, right?!" He laughed and laughed.

"Yes sir! That's me! That was my home group!" It was like a long lost brother coming home from war or something.

We talked for a few minutes about who we knew and who we were keeping in touch with and then I left him again. I came back a few more times to finish his admission and told him every time how I would take excellent care of him. Just like any good, sober alcoholic, he was always grateful and let me and the other staff know.

Despite the one good day in November, the month itself was still a shit show overall. After one confirmed and one presumed death, I concluded that statistically we weren't due for another death for at least a couple months. Wrong again…

Chapter 21

December

You win some. You lose some. - Bridget Delaney

November was gone and December came overnight. I heard all the holiday jingles on the TV from my med-cart in the hallway. Every ten minutes I heard Mariah Carrey's "All I want for Christmas." I thought about all the COVID outbreaks all over the country and how we could still be celebrating Christmas like nothing ever happened. I thought about all the Christmases with missing family members, who were deceased or in the hospital—and all the families who would be skipping Christmas entirely. Christmas was another holiday that my family and I missed, but we did manage to do an outdoor gift exchange around a fire. I remarked on how, during the actual plague, the king and some other royals would be on the inside of a ring of fire so the plague itself couldn't penetrate the circle of flames.

On December first, our census was around twenty-six, so we still had the two nurses and two CNAs. We had one resident whose mind was completely gone. She had a ten second goldfish memory. She would wheel herself out of her room without a mask and ask for cookies... every five minutes. Even if we gave her the cookies and her belly was full, her stomach didn't send the signal to the brain that she was full, and she kept asking for more cookies. After trying to talk to her and giving her cookies, I could only ignore her while I worked on more and more admissions. The nurses I worked alongside with were new RNs and didn't know how to do admissions. I tried to explain and teach what I could about the admission paperwork, but if they didn't do it themselves it was difficult to learn—like any new skill. On top of that, it was about the day's survival so I just hammered them out as quickly and thoroughly as I could, knowing that there were plenty of non-important documents I was neglecting. I taught the RNs, who were sometimes BSNs, all sorts of nursing tips, tricks, and skills. I thought them how to start IV solutions and manage IVs and the pumps that ran them. I retaught them how to draw and inject insulin the proper way. Apparently many nurses forgot these steps—it was still a wonder I remembered every step from seven years ago. I taught them G-tube tricks and how they weren't exactly approved protocol, but how it wasn't hurting the resident and was helping the nurse. I reminded them to auscultate bowel sounds before giving stool softeners or laxatives to ensure the bowels were working and there was no impaction, which in those cases would render the medication useless.

All the nurses I taught were grateful and one even gave me a Christmas gift. Her name was Monica and we worked for close to three weeks together. I taught her everything I knew and what was important and how to prioritize. She really appreciated it and let me know it every shift. She got me a big beautiful bag of chocolate with ribbons and a nice Christmas tree ornament, probably from some Martha Stewart collection, so you knew it was quality. When she gave it to me I faked great surprise and delight, but quickly lowered my head and began my acting bit, and said I was Jewish. Monica's smile evaporated before my eyes and a look of shock and terror took over. It looked like she was terrified of offending me. We stood there in silence looking at each other and then I said, "Just kidding! Thank you so much! This means so much to me!" We laughed and laughed and she told me how convincing I was. The truth was that I was really touched by her material reciprocation of my efforts with her. I felt like I did prepare her for her future jobs. When new nurses wanted to learn, I would teach them—just like Sarita did with everyone else. I wasn't eating any of my young, but rather nurturing and encouraging them. I wasn't exactly an experienced nurse and I probably shouldn't have been teaching anyone—after all, I was only ten months into my career, but I was one of the better ones in the facility after so many had left. Even if a nurse knew everything in every book written about nursing, the question was, did that nurse have the energy and desire to teach another human being everything they knew? Then *if* they did have the energy and desire to help teach other nurses, were they *good* at teaching?

I thought I was good at it and often pondered a career in teaching nursing. I would emphasize the reasons and rationale as to why we would do something—people remembered better if they knew the reason why it had to be such a way. I also hammered home the important parts with repetition, funny anecdotes, and instilling a fear of death as a consequence of silly mistakes: *too much insulin-ya dead! Too much anti-hypertensives- ya dead! Too much potassium-ya dead!* I tried to relate and make analogies that would help the student remember things better. Monica eventually went on to a hospital to do real work. I thought maybe we'd run into each other into the future. Monica was always grateful to learn and she worked very hard. Since I hadn't had a Christmas tree in years I gave the ornament to my regular CNA, Iris, when I saw her in passing in the hall as I left. You could give Iris Randall a paperclip and she would be happy and would think it was the darnedest thing. She loved free stuff. When the facility gave out tee shirts and I didn't want mine, she would tell me to hurry back and get one for myself so I could give it to her. She was grateful for the ornament. I wasn't sure if she thought I went to the store and saw it and thought—"Oh my! This is *so* Iris. She'll love this for a Christmas present." I never told her I'd regifted it. She never got that chocolate though, I ate all of it in less than three minutes. Certain self-control I still didn't have, especially when it came to sweets and delicious foods.

On nights where we had double admissions, the secondary nurse (yes, I named myself unofficial primary) would do most of the med-pass while I did paperwork at the desk. It was usually Monica and I and she had no problem doing the med-pass since that's what she knew and what she was comfortable with. I would run and help her with little things here and there but sitting down was good for my feet and legs. My newly developed varicose veins were creeping up my right leg and starting to throb. I had to believe standing on them in one place for eight hours had something to do with it.

Monica would come to the desk with questions and I would answer them. There weren't too many things I didn't know by this time. Most of the questions were about where to find something on the cart or what the medication's generic name was. By this time I knew dozens of medications—brand and generic, the form they came in, their purposes, as well as some side effects. I can recall phoning the MDs and going over the medication lists. I would tell them the medication and what it was for. We would speak in almost all medical terminology and I would comprehend all of it. I remember during one conversation stepping back and thinking to myself, "Wow! Maybe I really am a nurse? Or at least I could play one on TV with all these fancy medical words." It was sort of like an out-of-body experience of disbelief. Little did they know I was an alcoholic who'd just recently got his life together and who was now in charge of these patient's lives during a pandemic, relaying orders to doctors and teaching other nurses. Life certainly is funny and you could turn it around at any time. You just need to change your thinking, get some social support, and have a will to do so. Oh—and a belief, faith, and constant contact with God definitely helps.

During this time Vicky Fulton was now COVID negative and needed a floor where she would live the rest of her life. Since she was always yelling, the only appropriate room for her would be on 2B with the other scream queens. Rhonda Ford got discharged home in October to be with her husband. We were worried Rhonda wouldn't get the care she needed. After seeing her husband several times we all decided that he didn't really seem like a caretaker and got very frustrated with her in the ten-minute segments when he visited. We thought maybe he was into the monthly disability check he would be receiving, but I wasn't one to judge; instead, I prayed for them both. I wondered how Vicky would fit in as Rhonda's substitute. She would have an eerily similar response to the queens. She was much quieter once she arrived to the room of mayhem.

I got Vicky ready and wheeled her to the end of the hall towards the lobby. I forgot her face mask at first so I had to run the length of the football field one hundred-yard hall back to my med-cart and get her one, praying and hoping she wouldn't try to get up and walk in my absence. No one was allowed in the halls without one—no exceptions. I waited for ten minutes for the CNA from the second floor to come and get her. I piled her chart and other paperwork on her lap and started to sweat. I always had a sense of urgency, so waiting and doing nothing sent my anxiety soaring, in addition to my ever-perspiring skin under all the plastic PPE. I took the time to mentally prepare and organize my thoughts and priorities.

Around here I still had to make use of every minute I got. I prioritized the admissions in my head and would make a dent in them, then help Monica for a little bit, then get back to the desk. This would also help my legs—not standing or sitting too much at one time. Finally, the CNA came and picked her up, and wheeled her to the elevator. I'd already given report to the receiving nurse, but she seemed disinterested. She just had to give the resident her 2100 meds and nothing more. Vicky had already eaten and was in decent spirits. She wasn't yelling in the hallway—I guessed it was because the change in scenery she was taking in, distracted her. She had been confined to the same bed looking at the same ceiling for almost two weeks straight. I wished her luck and said farewell, not knowing if she could comprehend my salutations. I thanked the CNA and hustled back to my desk, reviewing my plan of attack in my head. Everything else went fine that night and we got through another night unscathed.

The next day we got a new admission, April Richards. She was a resident of our facility and she had already had COVID when it first hit so I thought she might be a false positive. I believed all the COVID numbers that were being reported had to have a good portion of their false positives. However, if someone tested positive we had to treat it like a real case and took no chances. April Richards was the one who was married on the front lawn of our facility. Her obesity, raging hypertension, diabetes, and congestive heart failure made her a perfect subject for the 'Rona reaper, so I knew I had to keep a keen eye on her. She and her husband spoke overnight through Skype on their computers. They loved telling us how expensive all their technology was. Her husband boasted about his printer in his room that never worked and how much money he spent on it. I figured I could get a better printer for fifty dollars. I wasn't sure if he got scammed into paying 150 dollars for it, or if he still thought 150 dollars was an exorbitant amount of money—either way, I pretended to be impressed by their electronic devices.

I tried to keep April happy and comfortable. She always liked me and preferred me to her other regular nurses. It was probably because I was able to get to everyone quickly and answered call bells within seconds. I was also very accurate when it came to medication administration and could name all six pills she was taking at the 1700 med-pass, and all nine pills she was taking at the 2100. She asked every night what each of them were.

During her time there, she constantly complained of pain in her back; she wasn't in her regular bed so I figured the pain may have worsened with the new sleeping arrangements. I gave her Tylenol around the clock. I constantly checked her oxygen. Sometimes her oxygen saturation would dip to ninety-one or ninety-two percent. I did my auctioneer bit for her. It was her first time seeing it and she thought it was hilarious. She laughed out loud, which actually helped her breathe a little better. I sat her up with her arms on top of the bedside table to improve her breathing. I told her to practice deep breathing to keep pneumonia at bay but I don't believe she ever did. She just said "yes" until I left. Her oxygen kept improving and worsening and whenever I was working I was sure to check on her at least once every half hour, for she was my most compromised resident.

April had been in the unit for about five days when her oxygen finally dipped below her previous low. She was eighty-nine percent so we put her on a nasal cannula at 2L per minute. Her oxygen shot up to ninety-four and ninety-five percent, but we were still worried. We had to check on her every fifteen minutes now. I could keep up the pace but I wasn't sure too many of my colleagues could do the same. Between forgetting about her altogether and doing the physical walking of fifty yards, it seemed unlikely. I remember her looking at me through her glasses while the nasal cannula made her uncomfortable, asking if she was going to die. This was the second time someone had asked me that, but my answer was the same: "What?! Don't talk like that! Come on now!" I didn't want to provide false hope but I also wasn't going to tell her that dying was a possibility. She seemed to be right in the eye of her own COVID storm and I hoped she would make it through the night. I knew her survival would depend on which nurses were on schedule for the next sixteen hours until I returned.

As I started to speculate which nurses might be coming to either stamp her death certificate or grant her more life, Sarita came bubbling through the double doors. Sarita could walk into a room and start a five-alarm fire with her presence alone—she could walk into the same room and put that same fire out just as easily. She was on a double shift and had just ended her first one as the 3-11 supervisor. She would now watch after half of our COVID patients. I told her that she would have to take the back side of the unit where our most serious patient was. I thought about God putting her in the right place at the right time. She told me how originally they

227

asked her to stay but her schedule wouldn't allow it, and then something opened up, permitting her to take the shift. I wondered if those strings were being pulled by the Big Guy himself.

I felt at ease leaving that night knowing that Sarita would kick COVID ass. If it were anyone else, I thought I might not ever see April again. Sarita was the closer coming in, in the bottom of the ninth, just like she had with Evelyn months before. We counted the narcotics and I gave her a report. Before I started the report I told her about April's condition and how she was a priority. I ended the report, saying the same. I felt stupid talking to a real live nurse like that but Sarita entertained my specific instructions and told me to get home safe. On the way out, I heard her directing the CNA to sit outside April's room all night with her chair facing the resident to report any difficulty breathing. I wished that one day I could be a confident, bad-ass nurse like Sarita. Maybe I would, but I would never acquire her fun Jamaican accent no matter how good a nurse I ever became.

When I got home, I watched replays from the Champions League in Europe. Weston McKennie and Christian Pulisic were playing for Juventus and Chelsea, respectively. I purchased special apps just to watch all their Champions League games. I followed MLS soccer religiously and only watched European soccer because of the American youth over there. I tried to savor the time away from my facility and enjoyed watching our boys in Europe. I kept thinking about April Richards and then told myself to stop thinking and stressing over it. I told myself I could do nothing about her situation while sitting in my apartment. I told myself that she was currently in the best hands and there was no better situation for her. I told myself to enjoy the day's matches that I'd missed. The fans were still absent because of Corona. I still couldn't escape the pandemic.

I was in an empty apartment watching soccer being played in empty stadiums. I felt empty without Shawna but tried to take solace in her cats. At least Moki was comfortable enough to sit on my lap while we watched our soccer. Keena was nowhere to be found. I wished she would love me like Moki did. I remembered my dad and how he'd said at least I had the cats to keep me company.

He was right, and I chose to be grateful that night. A brief gratitude list formed in my head… I was grateful I had these cats. I was grateful for Shawna. I was grateful for my health. I was grateful I had a career and was working. I was grateful for my sobriety and that I had my online Alcohol Support Groups to combat the pandemic of loneliness that accompanied COVID. I was grateful that I wasn't in April Richard's shoes...

...

The next day I came into the 1B COVID unit and immediately found that something wasn't right. There were two new BSNs, sitting around the desk with an air of anxiety about them. They looked relieved to see me and I asked what was the matter, worried. The one nurse Kelsey Madison said, "April's desatting to eighty percent and we can't get it any higher, she's on 10L per minute on a non-rebreather."

"Okay; EMS is on the way?" I asked calmly.

"No," she said casually. "We're waiting for a packet to put her paperwork in. We called 1A and..."

I interrupted her before she could finish as my body and mind entered panic mode and wished hers would do the same. "What?! Forget the paperwork! Call 911 right now!" I yelled as I dropped my backpack at the desk and hustled to April's room. I felt guilty about yelling but couldn't worry about her feelings at that moment. I thought about how I might have sounded like one of the nurses I despised. I didn't ever want to appear as though I was on a healthcare TV show putting people down when they made mistakes—but this was her ABCs—the most important three things in nursing; airway, breathing, circulation; and the resident wasn't breathing well. They should have acted sooner and better, but they were brand new nurses with not too many experienced nurses around to teach (or in this case, remind) them about priorities and fundamentals.

I got to the room and saw April laying almost flat in the bed and put her up to a sitting position. I put the bedside tray table in front of her and put her arms on top of it to open her lungs. I turned the oxygen up to 15 Liters and took the pulse ox from the bedside table to check her oxygen. (At least they'd kept the pulse ox in the room—that was a good move). I put the pulse ox on her finger and let it read the percentage. Seventy-nine percent was the new low. It teeter-tottered between seventy-nine and eighty-three even with the extra oxygen. I got another pulse ox using a different finger and then switched them around to confirm the instruments were working correctly. April could tell I was worried and asked me about dying again, I yelled, "Stop it, April, just keep breathing deep," and ran out of the room. Kelsey confirmed that EMS was on their way. As I walked to the phone I said, "Don't worry about the paperwork; ABCs are more important. She's not breathing well."

If April wasn't in the eye of the COVID storm last night, she certainly was now. Her lungs were working overtime to keep her alive and were beginning to fail. I paged overhead the in-house Nurse Practitioner who arrived on the scene minutes later. We both walked into April's room and stayed with her until EMS came. Kelsey filled in the EMTs on the way from the desk to the room. The nurse practitioner overheard Kelsey telling them that the oxygen had been dropping for the last two hours. The NP looked at me and rolled her eyes. It was a mistake to wait so long and in this situation mistakes were deadly. The two BSNs had six months of experience between them both and I ultimately blamed the staffing for this mistake. Often healthcare personnel don't ask for help, because they might appear weak or uneducated. It was ego and fear that drove these sorts of behaviors and decisions. Everyone was guilty of this, including me. I learned to shut my ego up most of the time and ask for help. If someone questioned my lack of knowledge, I would make a joke and say I was sleeping during that part of nursing school. I could also say, "Well, I'm not really a real nurse, I'm still learning." Maybe it was that fear of asking for help that kept April on our floor and out of an ER for a bit too long. Maybe it was just inexperience or laziness. I never questioned the nurses as to why they didn't send her out sooner or what exact moment they were waiting for.

EMS took her out on the stretcher. I walked with her for a bit down the football hallway and told her to hang in there, and that I'd let her husband, Perry, know that she was going out. The amount of oxygen she was receiving, her low oxygen saturation percentage, and all her diagnoses gave me an uneasy, nervous feeling. I called Perry and let him know the situation. I told him that she was having difficulty breathing and that the ER was the best place for her to be at the moment. We had no ventilators so if she needed one she could get one at the hospital.

I took report that evening an hour late and counted the narcotics. I reiterated the importance of the oxygen levels, especially during COVID wartime. I told them to consider where she was in the middle of the virus' course. She was around six or seven days since her positive test, which is when and where COVID would really hit—if it did at all. I confirmed that the reason for the delay was waiting for a special *envelope* with our letterhead to put the already prepared and organized paperwork in. I wanted to scream and punch a wall but held my anger and frustration in. I passive-aggressively asked them if it made sense to wait for an envelope when all the important paperwork was already gathered and prepared. The nurse confessed they never even confirmed the envelope was coming! They'd just left a message with someone on another floor! One of them started crying. I told her not to worry, and that this shit happens.

The two BSNs left and only I and the NP remained at the desk. The nurse practitioner was still very angry. She believed that they should have sent her out hours ago at the first sign of trouble, and let me know it. I agreed and countered with the fact that they were both inexperienced and had no help, despite their prestigious title and education. I tried to defend their lack of action and told the NP how both of them were hired in the summer and weren't even around during the first round of COVID. They were my buddies and I tried to teach them whenever I could but I just didn't work with them enough. She retorted that these were basic assessments and skills you learned in nursing school. She said that out of all the things you learn in nursing school, the ABCs and a handful of other information were the important ones that you just *can't* forget. We agreed that they should have known the resident was a full code status. This meant doing anything and everything to resuscitate a resident, and definitely send them out to the ER if she was having such trouble breathing. We agreed that they could have called the NP hours ago if they were unsure of anything.

The bottom line is that we don't know whether or not quicker decision-making and action could have saved April. It's possible that this second round of COVID was always going to be the one to bring her to her maker—no matter how quick we got her to the ER.

I like to think that I would have called EMS much sooner but I just don't know unless I'd been in that position and lived it. I know that Sarita must have given them a good report at 7 a.m. when she'd left. She must have told them to check on her frequently and check her oxygen levels as often. Maybe they got content towards the end of their shift and figured they would be escaping the game of Corona Roulette at 1500 when it was the next shift's problem.

Monica came in a little late so she missed all the chaos and commotion. We then learned we had two more admissions coming in so we split up the work between desk work and med-pass work like we often did. She still wanted nothing to do with the paperwork so she was happy with taking the cart. We banged out the 1700 med-pass together and quickly, as I waited for the new admissions. One came around 1800 and I started to get to work. I gave her simple tasks like rewriting orders on the physician order sheets once I confirmed them with the MD. This repetition would help her brain connect all 'five rights of medication administration' to writing them down on paper. Although she wouldn't write orders on paper after she left our facility, memorizing the 'five rights of medications administration' is vital in any area of nursing. Monica had already been interviewing with local hospitals so I wanted to prepare her the best I could—especially after thinking of me with that Christmas gift and all the gratitude she expressed daily.

We finished the admission and confirmed the pharmacy would be sending the medications that night. I helped her with the 2100 medications and we finished early. Around 2200, we waited anxiously for the next admission to burst through the COVID gates of hell. I imagined a hospital ER TV scene with doctors on either side of a stretcher accompanied by several EMTs pushing a stretcher quickly down a corridor. They would come to Monica and I to give report and we would save the life. That was a far cry from what was happening. We received stable residents who were just getting over COVID, so those types of scenes just didn't happen in our nursing home—but it could still be as hectic.

I reflected on the day and the April situation and said a quick prayer for her. I wondered why these nurses had been waiting on an envelope to put the paperwork in. When I questioned them about the envelope and what difference it would make, they had no answer so I figured they understood the lesson. It also perplexed me as to how they never confirmed an envelope was coming and how they left a message with another unit. I wondered how long they would have waited for that damn envelope if a change of shift hadn't come. I figured they'd learned their lesson after I yelled at them when I came on the unit. I imagined myself apologizing to them but also teaching them about what went wrong in that situation and what went right. In that same spirit of teaching, I recapped the situation with Monica and asked her if she would have waited for the envelope. She said she would have called 911. I told her how important breathing was and that when oxygen saturation reached below a certain level that you couldn't treat yourself, you had to call 911 and get them to a real hospital. She continued to agree and was also baffled by the delay. Her responses sounded good, but you just don't know how you'll act until you're in that situation yourself.

2300 came and Monica and I had dodged the roulette bullet. All the residents were safe and the new admission would be on the next shift's time so we didn't have to worry about it, which was an enormous relief. Monica remarked how she never got time to sit, never took breaks, and never even had time to go to the bathroom. She also commented on the fact that even though I took desk duties I still helped her with the med-pass.

She thanked me furiously. Most nurses who got assigned desk duties would rarely return to their feet to help other nurses on the med-carts— even if it was a slow shift and the desk nurse had nothing to do. Helping another nurse with their med-pass would be at the bottom of their non-existent to-do list. I liked Monica and didn't want to see her go. Our facility was a learning one. It was a stepping stone for nurses to gain six months of experience before they started a "real" nursing job in a hospital. Nursing home/long-term facilities were the double-A farm teams of nursing; and the hospital ERs, ORs and ICUs were the major leagues. I often expressed this sentiment to my nursing support group peers, but they always shut me down and told me that I need to give myself more credit and that I was indeed a real nurse! I imagined Monica in her new role, telling her coworkers that she learned all she knew from a kick-ass COVID LPN, but there go I and my delusions of grandeur. By now, I considered that my nine months of nursing in COVID wartime and the experience I had gained and all that I'd been through, might actually be the equivalent to three years of standard nursing. I was satisfied with that calculation and my confidence continued to grow.

…

It had been four days since we'd sent April out and the word was that she was on a ventilator and that her husband, Perry had been contacted about her condition. The hospital basically said they were going to keep her on the ventilator to see if she would rebound, and if that didn't happen that they would let her go. I'm not sure what Perry said or how he reacted, but April passed on two days after that call. The news hit everyone very hard. The whole facility, staff, and residents grieved for April; she was well-liked and was always participating in activities and making friends. In addition to her popularity, she had just gotten married on the front lawn of the facility so some of the residents could see from their rooms. Her recent nuptials made it even sadder for everyone.

I saw the NP almost daily and when she heard the news she practically blamed the new BSNs for the death and said that if they had reacted more quickly, the outcome could have been different. I didn't know if that was the case or if anything would have helped April, or if COVID would have taken her either way, but the NP was still angry. I wondered if she confronted the nurses. I never got the chance to apologize to the young BSNs or debrief with them. I saw them a couple more times in the coming weeks and our interactions were pleasant, but they went on to hospital jobs soon after. They would have an experienced nurse orienting and precepting them, and I knew they would gain the knowledge and skills they would need. Any weaknesses and knowledge deficits would be sniffed out by the experienced precepting nurse and would be remedied immediately. I was no one to judge and I hoped the best for them. I never got around to saying a prayer for them and their new career paths. Perhaps I'll do that now.

God, please bless Kelsey and Lana
Let them find their knowledge, strengths and wisdom on their path,
Please look after Kelsey and Lana and keep them safe,
Let them help many, if it is Thy will
Amen.

December brought another loss under my watch. It was an eighty-five year-old bed-bound man who was already awaiting death's arrival. He was more or less on hospice but since hospice nurses didn't come into the COVID units, he never was officially under hospice care. He stopped eating and drinking and taking his meds. It was only a matter of time, and the Covid roulette game started the day he arrived on the unit. He looked like death and smelled even worse. We could only make him comfortable. We brushed his gums with a foam-like swab to keep his mouth moist, and changed his briefs when needed. The day I lost the COVID roulette I had gone about two hours without checking on him. The CNA told me he didn't look well. I came in to find him deceased. His skin had turned a yellowish-green and there was no movement at all. I watched him for a full minute just in case; I didn't want to be the one to call the family and the funeral home only to find out he was just taking a nap. He was certainly dead. I went to call the family and found that he was a ward of the state, so I would notify the state's elderly guardian's office. They were probably getting dozens of phone calls a day during the second wave so I expected a quick conversation. Name, date of birth, time of death, okay thanks goodbye. The guardian wanted to know other specifics, which irritated me—I thought these questions were irrelevant and disrespectful to the deceased. I prayed for his soul and hoped he passed on to the other side easily and gloriously.

I had to call the funeral home and list the state's guardian's name and give some other information that the family of the deceased would normally do. They came and collected the body. This time the funeral home was prepared and had their n95. I got the undertaker a gown at the door and subtracted one soul from my census. We were having more discharges than transfers so our number was down to twenty. The majority of our cases were still recovering. I wondered when they would pull my second nurse and I would be alone again.

We had another resident from a sister facility who just couldn't beat COVID. His name was Clyde Doheny and his family was local and very much involved. I talked with them almost every night. He was another one more or less on hospice. I gave him morphine every two hours. After the previous death, I didn't worry about the paperwork or other labor that came with a death but decided to focus on the family and a peaceful passing for the resident. A wise nurse once told me that the way a person passes on is just as important as the life that person lived. The second day after he'd received the morphine order, I held it for a couple of hours until the daughter and son-in-law arrived at his window. I called them on my cell phone and put it on speaker so they could talk to him. The window blinds were open so they could see him, but the windows themselves were shut so the daughter and son-in-law were shielded from any droplets floating out into the cold winter air from his room. I left my phone and went about my 1700 med-pass. I checked back on them an hour later and the daughter was still saying things like "I love you," "It's okay to go," "We'll be all right," and "Thank you for everything." Too many times I had been in charge of residents who were unable to say goodbye to their families and died alone, so I decided this passing was a win for myself as I cried quietly outside the door. I thought my tears wouldn't flow anymore due to my calloused heart after all the wreckage of the COVID, but this goodbye brought them back like a river pouring through a broken dam.

The family saw me and waved me in. I didn't have time to pull myself together and entered the room as soon as they beckoned me. My adrenaline stopped my tears altogether, but the daughter could still see the redness and swelling in my eyes and no doubt put two and two together. They thanked me profusely and said their final goodbye. I vigorously sanitized my phone and left it on the cart open to the air. I gave the resident his long-overdue morphine. He passed away less than a half-hour after that. The daughter was still on the road when she got my phone call. I told her how sorry I was for her loss, but how grateful I felt that they got to say goodbye, as so many others before him didn't get that chance. I cried some more and maybe she knew it or maybe she didn't, but she thanked me so much again. I told her that she had to call the funeral home to make funeral arrangements and pick up the body. *How awkward.* That was the last time I spoke with Clyde's daughter. The funeral home courier came and I sent another body out. I thanked God for the goodbye they'd shared and the smooth, swift passing that followed.

...

Nate Ranieri was another resident successfully discharged at the tender age of ninety-one. He lived at home with his wife. They were both independent but had their sons and grandchildren in the area to check on them a couple of times a week. When he was still with us, he was always irritated at the situation but always made jokes, which I loved. We talked about Italian football and he told me his team was Napoli. They were a mid-table team in *Serie A* but we shared a connection through soccer.

I paid extra special attention to the cases that would be discharged back to independent home life. I felt like their lives mattered more than those who would go back upstairs or to another nursing home. All lives were equal in through a nurses eyes, but I thought my work meant more to someone who had a life to get back to.

I talked with one of his sons every evening and gave him his updates. Apparently, I was the only one in the facility they were in contact with regarding his father's care, and he was grateful for the time I took and thanked me before and after each conversation. He also knew not to keep me on the phone for too long because of how busy we were, and was content with my brief updates. Nate complained about missing Christmas and how much it meant to Italian families. I told him how many holidays I had missed and he told me that I had him beat. He got out a couple of days before Christmas came, and he and his family were delighted. I got to meet the son I'd spent two weeks talking to every night, and he also thanked me for a job well done. We stood at the COVID gates as I handed Nate off to his son, in his wheelchair. Our eyes met and he thanked me and I said "Molto Bene! Ciao familia! Forza Napoli."

Nate said in his Italian accent, "We a' gonna send you a' some a' fish on a' Christmas Eve!" We all knew he was kidding and we all laughed as they left through the lobby back to a semi-normal, freer life.

. . .

Christmas eve saw our census at thirteen and that was the magic number—I would no longer be receiving an extra nurse and CNA. I did my best and the admissions continued to slow down. Residents were getting out sooner than the standard two-week quarantine. If residents were asymptomatic and tested negative for the virus, they could leave as soon as ten days. The last week-and-a-half, we discharged or transferred most of the last thirteen residents.

Two days after Christmas and one day before Shawna's arrival back home from her last travel assignment, her Christmas gift arrived and was installed and mounted. It was a seventy-inch smart TV. We'd had an older TV since we moved in and desperately needed an upgrade. The folks from

Best Buy came in and installed it in less than twenty minutes, and it was perfect. In anticipation of her return, I kept telling her how I bought her such a big gift. She was a good guesser but never figured out what it was until she walked into the apartment and saw it. In my head I played the scene dozens of times, but I never got the big red bow that would make it extra special. She loved it all the same.

She was home for four days, and would fly out on December thirty-first back to California for her next assignment. She would be stationed at The Fairgrounds in the San Jose area doing drive-through COVID swabbing. Everything was drive-through now!

We spent our short time together and I had to share the time with her two cats that she adored and missed terribly. Moki and Keena slept in the crevice of her legs and near her face every night. By the time Keena, the handicapped kitten, warmed up to her and got reacquainted with her rescuer, Shawna was on the plane and gone the next day.

Chapter 22

January

Happy New Year and Happy Homecoming!

Everyone in the world was ready for the new year. I only did one week in January on the COVID floor before it was closed and terminally cleaned. We had fancy new UV ray machines that would kill the virus as soon as the light hit it. I never saw these devices but had to believe in them. Everything would be bleached and the windows opened for a week to ensure a clean unit. I left the unit around January eighth and returned to my home on 2B. It was my second homecoming in less than a year. I'd done two COVID tours of duty and wondered if this was how military personnel felt coming home. Although there were some similarities, I decided I couldn't compare it to live combat.

Everyone was happy to see me. Some of the residents knew where I'd been the whole time. Other residents thought I'd quit or gotten fired. Some staff members actually thought I was a traveler and had left because my assignment was over. Wally Lasiter joked and said he thought the virus took me. We laughed about it and I told him I was happy to see him. I told Jim Moss that we had a lot of singing to make up for, and he agreed. I sang "Back in Black," by ACDC, even though I was in my classic navy blue scrubs. I walked out and kept listening to him screeching the lyrics. Boy, it was good to be home.

I checked on all my residents and some were generally more chatty than others. They wanted to know what the virus was doing and who was infected and who had survived. I told them that that information was confidential and above their pay grade. Some of them laughed and others agreed that they didn't want to know. Some just didn't get the joke.

After a week of being back, I noticed that Leslie wasn't trying to walk at all. Her legs were probably so weak that even her disheveled mind knew well enough that her legs would not carry her weight anymore. She had gained a few pounds which further complicated her ambulatory skills. There was decline in all the residents all over the facility.

Corey Chapman used to be able to stand on two feet and turn a little bit to get in and out of bed, but now he would require a mechanical lift to accomplish that task. Finding the lift, confirming its battery was charged, and then transferring an extra-large resident in it was an operation in and of itself, so it was difficult to get him out of bed, especially when we had skeleton crews working the unit. I actually saw a CNA tell Jeoffrey Pratt to go get Corey out of the bed with the lift. I'm not sure if she knew Jeoffrey was a resident and not an employee.

Corey became aggravated easily but I took this opportunity to try and motivate him to lose weight. I told him if he could drop all the extra pounds, walking again would be a possibility. I also told him how unhealthy it was to be that obese and of the risks it brought. He cut out all juice that he used to drink with each meal, watched his portions, and really started to exercise with Luna and the gang. He would lose over twenty-five pounds in the next couple of months. He was excited when they weighed him each month and couldn't wait to tell me the new number and the new low he achieved. I told him that *work is never over* and that this was just the beginning. I told him to lean on Luna and others who were exercising and trying to eat healthy. I told him to talk to others about his eating and exercise. I mentioned how I used social support every day to keep my mind and body healthy and how the same principles applied here. He was mentally challenged after all, so I wasn't sure if he truly grasped the principles and suggestions I gave him.

Luna was still kicking butt and was happy to see me back on the floor. She was one of the few who could actually verbally express how happy and grateful she was to have me back. She had a new roommate and was taking care of her the best she could. If she wasn't rubbing lotion on her roommate's swollen legs, she was helping her with basic activities of daily living. Luna would order coloring books and crayons for her new roommate to keep her busy. Luna and her roommate both came from living at home independently so they shared a similar story and frustration about being locked up in a nursing home.

I checked on Vicky and the other two scream queens. Just like Rhonda Ford, Vicky lost her voice once she moved into the corner quad room. Jan Konkle and Leanne Donovan would yell all day long and I guess Vicky just couldn't keep up the pace. I learned that Vicky liked it when I would dance or do a jig. I did simple box steps that I remembered from my high school musical production of "George M." It made her smile and maybe she escaped her prison quarters for a moment. She would swing her arms about in response to my dancing, almost like Carlton from the *Fresh Prince of Bel Air*. This simple dance number allowed me to give her one scoop of applesauce and medicine. After the first spoonful she would start yelling and throwing her arms about to keep me from giving her more. I had to cram all six of her crushed pills into one small amount of applesauce. This was a quirk I had to learn about her, just like I did with all the other residents. Preferences, do's and don'ts. I thought that it must have tasted terrible and was grateful I was the one on the other side of the spoon. As the sun went down though, she became more and more irritated and would refuse her vital signs checks and later medications.

My unit had received several new residents since my two-month COVID tour. One was Jeoffrey Pratt who I had spoken to a handful of times and tended to like. The other thing about him was, he got way too close physically and had no sense of personal space. I would continuously back up and move out of his way but he never could take the hint. He used to be a construction worker and basically functioned on the unit as an extra CNA. He would also fix TVs and tray tables and drawers and beds, so that won him the title of Maintenance as well. He was a huge help and I was grateful to take care of him now. I was extra thankful when I flipped to his Medication Administration Record pages and saw that he took only two medications and neither were on my shift! This was the ideal resident! I wished for twenty-seven more just like him!

I did whatever favors I could for Jeoffrey because he was such a big help. He was constantly getting residents water and clearing their lunch and dinner trays. Once he was allowed out of his room it was like he had to make up for lost time. He worked harder than anyone else in the building and was still our most valuable *CNA*. I wished I could give him medications to dish out up and down the halls, but that would spell disaster and if anyone saw it I would surely be fired! He liked to eat and he loved his soda so I always made sure to get him his signature Mountain Dew whenever I was at the corner store. It was my form of payment for his day-to-day service to others. He was always grateful and thanked me. Another cheap way to make someone's day. How could I pass it up?!

The other new resident was Lennie Barker. He was another aphasic resident secondary to stroke secondary to hypertension secondary to drug/alcohol abuse. The only words he could say were *truth, love,* and *uh-huh!* If he had pain he would have to point to the area and we would use the Wong-Baker FACES scale to determine the amount of pain he was in. He was on minimal medicine as well, but instead of helping residents he would wander into residents' rooms and open drawers and cabinets. He would touch people who didn't want to be touched, and would sometimes playfully slap staff members on the arms or back. He was a nuisance because of his behavior but he was quite lovable. He had a high-pitched laugh that you could identify from thirty yards down the hall. His laugh made *you* laugh… or at least smile.

He never helped others but he was good at keeping some folks company, particularly Anita Gregg. She spoke only Spanish and he couldn't speak anything other than his three catch phrases, but they would still have hour-long conversations on the hot corner. Every five minutes, they would burst out in laughter and we all wondered what they could be laughing about. Lennie and Anita would go on walks all the way down the football hall and beyond to the other side of the facility and back. Anita used a cane and the waist-high bumper rails lining the walls of the corridors, but when she had Lennie she would hold his one good arm and they would walk at a slow pace. It was adorable to watch and everyone loved to see it. It was a relationship no one would ever understand but its foundation was friendship.

Jim, Wally, and Frank Dusen were all still roommates and nothing had changed much in their lives. Jim still never got out of bed. Wally still loved his sports and puzzles and some quick wit. Frank slept a lot and would continue to steal employees' food out of the staff refrigerators when he wasn't sleeping. Wally and Jim were happy to have me back and they both told me how they'd missed me, and how they weren't sure I was ever coming back. The thought of leaving everyone had made me sad, but the fact that some remembered me and told me so, must have meant I was doing something right.

Next to the quad rooms and across from my 2B desk was Tabatha Pattersons's room. Ruby Vedder was now on hospice and had moved to a private room at the beginning of the football hallway. Tabatha was alone in her room for a couple days and dreaded another noisy roommate. Ruby and her Silent Night on repeat had ruined the song and probably the holiday altogether for Tabatha.

The new roommate was Thuy, the forty-three year-old Vietnamese stroke victim I'd cared for on the quarantine unit during my last tour. She'd been Vicky Fulton's COVID roommate. Thuy was a cosmetologist/manicurist and had no healthcare. She was a charity care case. I presumed she never had insurance and never had seen a doctor which is why she hadn't known about her hypertension. In her case there were no drugs or alcohol to exacerbate the hypertension but it was there nonetheless and had caused a stroke and a brain bleed. She was probably 4'11" and weighed a hundred pounds. She spoke broken English but could say the three most important words in the English language: "Please," and "Thank you." She was always so kind and grateful for whatever you did for her. Because of her attitude of gratitude she won the hearts of all the staff and residents, including her crabby ninety-year-old roommate Tabatha.

"Oh... I... just... love her!" Tabatha said slowly to me when I asked how her living situation was going.

"That's good Tabatha, I'm glad."

"She's... so... sweet... I... just... love her! " she reiterated to me and everyone else who asked.

Later on I saw Tabatha doing little things for Thuy, who preferred to stay in bed. Staying in the wheelchair for more than half an hour would tire Thuy out quickly. Tabatha often remarked that having Thuy was like having a daughter or granddaughter to look after. This was just what Tabatha needed—service to others and a purpose. Tabatha had more pep in her step since Thuy moved in. It was almost annoying when Tabatha would chime in to let staff and other residents know what Thuy's preferences were and how to care for her. Thuy would roll her eyes when

Tabatha couldn't see them and we would have a secret laugh about Tabatha, the newly promoted guardian and watchdog. Tabatha would also feel some sort of way when Luna would come in and sing "you are my sunshine" with her. Eventually everyone on the hot corner would sing the song together at least once a day.

I could be having the worst day ever and then after helping Thuy with something and receiving her dozens of thanks, be in the best mood ever. I would get my second wind from her and be re-energized as if I had just started my shift. Thuy had a positive effect on everyone she encountered.

Brenda still liked to watch my six, but she could only hang for shorter amounts of time now and it took her longer to catch up to my med-cart when she wheeled herself to my location. She would often fall asleep right in the hall and we would have to put her to bed earlier than she wanted.

Lucie Greer, Brenda's roommate, who also had a parental role was able to alert staff when Brenda wasn't looking good or was in pain. Lucie would always give me report each evening as to how much Brenda ate at breakfast and lunch. She would also do her best to tell me how much water she was drinking. I joked and told her not to be late to our 1800 briefing each night. She was in bed by 1600 so she wasn't going anywhere anyway, but she loved my jokes and was one of the few who actually understood them.

Being back on my unit got me thinking about how we could film a TV show up here and how certain residents would be recurring characters, each with their own catchphrases: Jordan Cliff's signature, "I don't give a fuck!" Leanne Donavan predictable, "That… tastes… TERRIBLE!" The late Barbara Watkins's smiling and high-pitched "AIGHT!"—although, it would be a sad episode when she passed away. And Anita Gregg's frustrating, yet lovable, "COMO?!" These folks could be stars!

The rest of the residents were more or less about the same as I'd left them. Randy Bahler had moved down to a single room towards the end of the hall. He was my resident here and there because he had the first room down the football hallway. He was in a double room but was the only occupant because of his bipolar and paranoid schizophrenic diagnoses. He was a very large man which made him a candidate for living alone. If he stopped taking his medications or had a bad day his temper and body might do a lot of damage to a smaller elderly person. He was fully mobile and I guessed he could probably bench press 250 without any practice. He was probably about the same size as Ben Roethlisberger.

I always tried to keep him happy because I didn't want to be on the receiving end of some violence that he could dish out. We were never able to establish a real rapport but he always remembered me and thanked me when I cared for him. He had a low-pitched, nasally voice and would ask me for cookies every night; "Got any cookies?" I always got him those cookies and darn quick. He shared his cookies with Anita on the hot corner for a couple of minutes once Lennie left his seat next to her.

Another resident we received from another unit was Henry Potter. He was Jamaican and lived towards the monster desk in the middle of the facility. He moved down the street and around the corner to the back of my forty-yard hallway. We had a couple vacancies since our former residents had been taken by the virus, and administrators were trying to pair up whoever they could to open up more rooms in the facility. Henry was wise and turned out to be very sweet. Henry and Luna became friends through food. Henry was the first stop on the snack train and he never forgot it. He ate whatever Luna gave him and was grateful. When Luna was sent to the hospital one week, the day she returned Henry stayed with her the whole day to make sure she was okay. I'm not sure if any food was exchanged but Luna told me this and it warmed both our hearts. I always liked Henry and when I heard this I liked him even more.

I had to take care of the residents who took care of all the other residents. Residents like Jeoffrey Pratt and Luna Wolfe were my top priority when it came to extras and favors that they needed. When I wasn't around the residents generally had to fend for themselves and take care of each other. As unfortunate and unfair as it was, that was the situation they were in. I decided younger generations wouldn't and couldn't be as tough as these generations. Every generation got softer and softer and I imagined they would crack once they found themselves in a nursing home with no help. I felt privileged to be taking care of those from some of the greatest generations our country has ever seen.

The oldest resident I cared for was ninety-nine at the time. I wished I could sit and listen to all of their stories, but the sad truth was that there was absolutely zero time for any walks down memory lane. Any time someone would start on a story, that anxiety and sense of urgency would kick in. I'd be so worried about falling behind I'd hardly retain anything they said. Sometimes if I didn't want to be rude, I would poke my head out of their room and into the hallway and shout, "Okay, I'll be right there!" knowing that the resident story teller couldn't hear well enough to know I was actually bluffing. One day, Henry caught me responding to the ghost staff in the hallway, figured out my bluff, and laughed hysterically, which I thought was hilarious. Henry knew well enough to keep my secret. He was smooth and keen like that and now I liked him *even more.*

Some of the residents I would pick up on short-staffed days would think I was a doctor. They were stuck in the thinking from decades ago that females had to be nurses and males had to be doctors. If a resident was cognitively sound I would explain who I was and what my duties were. For others it made no sense to try and explain that I was a nurse and not a doctor. Some residents would even take their medication easier if they thought the doctor was in! They had the utmost respect for doctors and would listen to them, more often than nurses.

I continued to entertain everyone as best I could and provide the best care possible. Lucie, Corey, and Luna asked for Shawna every day and asked where she was. I told them every day that she was still in California doing drive-through COVID swabs. I told them how she and her team were responsible for thousands of COVID tests each day. I showed them pictures she sent me on my phone of the long lines of cars in the beautiful park. The weather was chilly in that part of California so she had to stay bundled up all day long. It was easy work, but it was still standing on your feet for eight hours in the brisk weather. The money was well worth it.

It was official that February first we would transfer ownership to a new for-profit health care company. Everyone was worried that staffing and resources would get worse. We speculated that certain fat might get trimmed and we'd be losing a lot of employees because of the new company's money-making mindset. I tried sharing my ideas on speculation and how worthless it was, but everyone preferred to talk about the unknown anyway. I'm not sure if it made them feel better, or if maybe through gossip they thought they could figure it all out before it ever happened. I told my colleagues no matter what, we'd still be here taking care of our residents and that nothing would change. One CNA said, "… unless they fire us all! Then what?!"

I laughed out loud as obnoxiously as I could in her face and joked how no one wanted to work here which is why we were always short-staffed and how job security would be a non-issue. I reminded her how she was in the union and how we were practically invincible. I shouldn't have said that last part in case she already didn't believe that about her union—this might have made her more inclined to underperform.

The other big news was the availability of the vaccine to all of us "Health care heroes." Leave it to New Jersey's governing bodies to make a mistake on the federal government's paperwork needed to get New Jersey facilities the vaccines. Whatever clerical error that was made, caused a two-week delay in our receiving the vaccine.

Chapter 23

February 2021

Life comes full circle!

Shawna came back in early February for the whole month, before her next assignment would begin. Since the vaccine was finally available, she looked for jobs administering the vaccine and would choose the highest bidder. She eventually chose to go to back to California. This time it was San Francisco. She was stationed at Levi Stadium, home of the San Francisco Forty-Niners. She would be a monitoring nurse and not actually administer the vaccine. Her job was to watch a dozen people for fifteen minutes at a time to make sure they had no adverse reactions. She enjoyed the easy job and only had to take care of one person who fainted after receiving the shot. The person was fine and she went about her day, continuing her assignment.

February first was a weekend and a bad snowstorm. I worked that Saturday with no one else, it seemed. No one could make it to work because of the snow. Since our new apartment was next door to the facility, I showed up on time and ready for work. When the new administrator made it in, he saw that I was there plugging away, and thanked me for showing up. I hoped this would win points with the new company, or maybe more money… I soon learned it would do nothing for these greedy geriatric generals. I figured this start to the new for-profit era was a bad one, and maybe was indicative of how things would go in the future.

I was able to get my vaccine in the first week of February. I hoped everyone would shut the fuck up about COVID. I knew my parents and siblings would be more open to me visiting my nieces and nephews and grandfather once I was fully vaccinated. There were about six or seven employees from the local CVS in the facility's dining room administering the vaccine. We would check in at the first booth, double-check our information, present our ID, then go to the next booth where we'd actually receive the shot. The dining room was full for about two hours at the 1500 change of shift for the week that the pharmacy occupied it. The Director of Nursing came in to see a full dining room and a line out the door. She said, "Wow! Look at this! I'm very happy to see all of you up here!"

"Nano-chip micro trackers, here we come!" I yelled out. Some people laughed, I didn't look to see the Director of Nursing's facial reaction, but she laughed out loud and thanked all of us for coming.

It took me no time at all to realize that everyone—including the Director of Nursing—was worried about the vaccination rate and the anti-vaxxers and the possibility that we would never turn the COVID corner. The anti-vaccine community and their opinions and thoughts were all over social media and even the regular media. People wanted their freedom and their choice in getting the vaccine. Many wanted no part in mandated vaccines. As a nurse, I wanted to do my part and get the vaccine that could end COVID, and also to show others that I was still alive and breathing, even after receiving the vaccine.

That same day I got to my unit at 15:30. *Already Late!* I got report from Jenny who was a brand new LPN. It turned out she would be taking over the regular 7-3 shift after Tanya had transferred to couch duty and unemployment. Jenny was twenty-two years old and had the ability to work hard. Her nurse's brain wasn't fully developed yet, so she missed a lot of silly stuff. She was also guilty of something I'd often seen the younger population doing to anyone and everyone. It seemed when a person had a question or an issue, the Gen-Z youngster would say anything to shut you up and move on from the conversation. They didn't realize that they could be held accountable for their words and actions in the future! If they did realize it would come back around, I guess they figured they would deal with it then… Either way, Jenny was a good nurse and followed through on most things. I found her guilty of this offense one too many times but never called her on it. Maybe my generation was also guilty of this, but I don't remember telling someone some bullshit just to shut them up and have them on their way and out of my face. I found Jenny making up policies and rules and telling residents about the fictitious laws to get her way in that moment. Then, when the residents questioned someone else about Jenny's made up policy, we responded the best we could— usually baffled!

One thing Jenny did that was funny, was telling the residents "Let's have a moment of silence," while she attempted to obtain blood pressures. I thought this was very clever for the Gen-Z nurse who was always stuck on her phone. I had a similar technique although not as clever. When taking blood pressures I would say one of two things—or maybe both. "Be still like a statue!" and I would freeze while trying to encourage them to do the same. With Corey, I would say, "Don't move. Don't talk. Don't touch!" If he kept talking I would say something like, "Zip that lip, Chip!" Sometimes they would listen and other times they wouldn't. Between Jenny and I, we needed to communicate and work well together to give our residents the best care.

I took report from Jenny and was not impressed. I remembered my first report, so I cut her *tons* of slack slack. Life had come full circle for me, and I had to give to newcomers so freely what had been given to me, *exactly* like Alcohol Support Groups taught me. All the Alcohol Support Group's principles were present in my life outside of the rooms. I asked her some important questions about residents. On questions she couldn't answer, I told her why they were important. She answered other ones skillfully. We flipped through the paper report and I saw she had drawn stupid little hearts all over. I decided to let it go, but it certainly got to me.

We counted the narcotics on the cart and I explained to her why we counted it and how to do it. Apparently whoever had been counting with her for the first month of her career had been doing it wrong. I approached her as if it was her first time. I could tell she wanted to scream at me, "I know what I'm doing! What the fuck?!" I got to the last page and noticed another one of her fucking hearts. "Jenny, what is this?" I stared at her as hard as I could, hoping I would burn through her eyes and out of the back of her skull with imaginary laser beams.

She cocked her head to the side, took a step towards the narcotic book, and began to scan the page, looking for what I was talking about. "What is what? There's eight tramadol left."

I couldn't tell if she was being smart, playing dumb—or if she was actually just dumb.

"The hearts, Jenny. Please stop doing that shit. This is a legal document and part of this resident's health information. Don't put hearts anywhere on these papers. And while we're at it please keep your signatures and initials in your own box. Your 'J' goes down into all my boxes all the time, and it's a pain in the ass for me to sign. Otherwise, good job. Keep it up." I walked around back to the desk and got on the phone before she could respond. I decided to give her the old compliment sandwich so I didn't hurt the snowflake's feelings too bad. I also didn't want to become the nurse who ate their young. I've been on the other end of that, and it's very frustrating and doesn't do anything but create resentments, and resentments were dangerous.

As I was beginning my 1700 med-pass I saw a figure walking down the football hallway. It was Sarita and I knew she had bad news for me.

"'Ey Papa! 'Ow you doing?" she said, bubbly and animated, leaving no time for me to answer the rhetorical question. "Papa dere's only two o' you. You 'gone be fine doe. Cathy countin' 'dat utta cart no problem. I'll see you later." She walked away.

She knew this news would ruin any nurse's day as it began, but also knew there was nothing she could do about it. Sarita was the type of supervisor who would take the cart for the shift, but her busy schedule probably didn't permit it that night. I wanted to huff and puff and yell and scream and kick and punch walls but all that, as always, would get me nowhere. I decided to accept it as fast as I could and get done with everything as fast as I could. On short-shifted days, we weren't nurses. We were pill passers. No time for assessments and real nursing duties. Just get the pills down the throats—or G-tubes—and try to make sure no one fell or choked on something.

Although I hated having the extra dozen residents, I did get to interact with new people and tried to connect with them as best I could. A lot of times I didn't have the time to have a genuine conversation, but I did get to know one resident who would become one of my favorites. Her name was Delilah Merton. I had taken care of her before, but had never gotten to really connect. She had a bobblehead of Noah Syndergaard that I had never noticed before, and that was all we needed for common ground. We talked about the Mets every time I came to give her medicine. On top of the New York Mets connection, she was absolutely colorful and entertaining. She had severe anxiety and tried to talk as fast as her thoughts would run in her head, but could never keep up. Before she would ask a question she would have to tell me about the question and present the reasons as to why she had to ask the question. She would add disclaimers about how busy I was but how she still just *had* to ask the question. She would apologize in advance for asking the question and for interrupting my duties. I would start laughing in her face to which she often took offense, but it was still just the funniest thing. I would finally say, "Delilah! Just ask!"

She would then say flustered, "Okay, okay. I'm sorry. I just didn't want to..."

"Spit it out!" I chuckled as I raised my voice a little bit, not wanting her to think I was mad at her. She would probably lose sleep over it. I imagined her lying in her bed, living in her head thinking about our *confrontation* that didn't really happen. She was sweet but spastic and unpredictable. She was the clumsy person who was always hurting herself by accident. She would bump into furniture and drop her water daily. She would turn her head so violently and quickly that her glasses would go flying to the floor. I would try to tell her to calm down but it usually never worked. She could not comprehend the word *relax* or the phrase, "Take it easy." One night I had nine of her pills ready to go. I walked into the room, confirmed she had enough water to drink with them, and placed the medicine cup in her hand. I should have told her to focus on the pills in hand, because she started to tell me something, using her hands to make gestures, and as she did all the pills went flying out of the cup. I laughed loudly because it was too damn funny not to, and I couldn't stress that I would have to prepare all nine pills all over again—plus there was no narcotics in the cup so I didn't have to get on my hands and knees looking for a controlled drug. Luna and Delilah were also becoming friends, which may have been a reason I took an extra interest in Delilah. We are all still friends to this day. Luna and Delilah exercise together and listen to a lot of Mets games on the Audacy App on Luna's iPad.

I also got to know Josh Lemon who's brain had been completely ruined with dementia. He was another ten-second Tom. He was also another cookie monster. He was also another person who liked to enter residents' rooms without permission and proceed to touch people... without their permission. He was pleasant most of the time but I didn't need an extra resident causing trouble around my unit who wasn't legally my responsibility. He would always come looking for cookies and I would indulge him when there were cookies to be found. To prevent him from entering my area I would turn my cart horizontally, making a blockade that he couldn't get around. I would distract him other times. And sometimes I would trick him, "They're looking for a Josh Lemon," while peering over his head down the football hallway, "Are you Josh Lemon?"

"Yea! What's it to you, Kemosabe?" He got excited and started to turn where I was looking.

"They need Josh Lemon down there, something about a cookie convention," I said, trying not to laugh.

"Alright, I know what they want. I'll go and take care of it." He sighed and wheeled towards the 2C mega desk. "See ya later alligator," he said to me with his back turned, and then responded to his own farewell, "After a while, croc of shit!" This got me laughing. I turned around and saw Jordan Cliff looking at me with skeptical eyes. I said quietly to him, "Got that sumbitch good!"

He let out a boisterous laugh and we shared a moment... although it may have been at the expense of someone else. I didn't want Lemon on my unit disturbing the peace and figured it was okay to keep him occupied with finding the fictitious cookie-con, at least until he forgot about it.

Towards the end of February, I got my second dose of the vaccine. It felt like I had the flu. It only lasted for about twenty-four hours. The night I got the dose I was shivering violently in bed and at one point I remember thinking it could be the end for me. After the moments of self-pity and morbid thinking, I decided to let go and let God decide my fate. I decided my faith in God and God himself would take care of me—whatever the outcome. I fell asleep shivering violently with extra blankets on top of me.

...

I woke up the next day and felt like I had been hit by the same hangover truck that would always get me after every night of drinking for the decade prior. I never even considered going to work and called out as soon as I got out of bed. I was in no condition to work. The chills were accompanied by a headache that made my brain feel like a swelled birthday balloon. A general feeling of lethargy and aches went along with my other symptoms, but I still felt terrible for notifying my work of the sick day I needed to take. I think the physical illness I was feeling was only slightly worse than the guilt I felt for my comrades because they would no doubt be short for my shift. The only silver lining was that I was fully vaccinated!

The whole month of February we worked short. Literally every other shift I worked I had to pick up an extra dozen residents. It was like the first two weeks of COVID all over again, minus the head-to-toe PPE. It was absolute hell, and just like that first two weeks of COVID, I was able to organize, prioritize and reacquaint myself with the assignment and its residents. I imagined myself in a montage, as I got faster and faster and it became second nature again. I was able to do little things here and there for the residents to try and really care for them.

Each night I got home and told Shawna whether I was short or not. On the days I was, she would scoff and roll her eyes and tell me about Texas law not allowing a nurse to take more than twenty long-term residents. I told her how nice that idea sounded, but how it would never happen in Dirty Jersey. She asked me where our union was when all this type of stuff happened. I had no answer for her. I told her we should be receiving time-and-a-half when we had to pick up another half an assignment. That seemed reasonable though I never presented it to the new company. They were unapproachable and if you did get them to listen, they would yes you to death and tell you they'd look into it. Money was their bottom line, not safety or quality of care.

During this time (and even to this day) the weekend shifts were absolute hell. The staff enjoyed their every-other-weekend off, took time to rest and see family and do whatever else, and they absolutely looked forward to it. For the residents, it was entirely the opposite. They dreaded and feared the weekends. They knew what was in store for them. Most of the residents would lay in their beds for the whole forty-eight hours because of staff shortages. There were not enough CNAs to get anyone out of bed on the weekends. The CNAs would have anywhere from twenty to thirty residents and all they could do was make sure every resident ate their meals and were changed once during their eight-hour shift. I felt terrible for my residents, but there was not much I could do aside from showing up an hour early to get a handful of residents out of bed and into their wheelchairs. I had never considered anyone anywhere ever disliking weekends, but this was the population who absolutely loathed Saturdays and Sundays for the worst reasons. Neglect and abandonment are probably the worst things a human could go through aside from physical pain and torture.

With all the extra residents and the slack the nurse had to pick up due to the shortage of CNAs, I started to incorporate a strategy I learned from Shawna and her med-pass. During the first hour and a half, when it was too early to start passing the 1700 medications, and after checking on all the souls on the manifest to make sure they were safe and accounted for, I would prepare every medication I planned to give during that eight-hour shift. I spent the first two hours flipping through the pages of the Medication Administration Record and putting pills in cups and organizing them. I would write the names of the residents on the plastic or paper medicine cups as well as the times of administration. The shallow top drawer of my med-cart was filled with dozens of medicine cups holding hundreds of pills. This was not allowed in nursing, or at least was frowned upon, and I never inquired as to the legality of this strategy. I reasoned that they were *still* in no position to fire nurses for silly offenses like pre-popping medications. Nursing rationale would state that this way of doing things would lead to medication errors. The nurse was supposed to do each resident and their respective medications one by one. I figured if I could do it safely and label the medications and be careful about it, I could lower the risk—I was also the regular nurse for the floor so I knew everyone and their medications much better than a substitute nurse. I compared the nursing rationale and "laws" to what I thought God would think about my new time-saving technique. I thought the Big Guy wouldn't mind—after all, doing it this way was a *time saver* and I could take better care of everyone with the extra time I had.

I asked my familial nursing panel about the unfair assignments on our group text, *Shift Report*. My older sister replied via text: "No one cares. Work harder." She elaborated that nursing was full of unfair assignments and duties and we could only do our best and work hard. My little sister replied by text: "That's not right. Tell them you refuse the assignment." I practically laughed out loud at her suggestion, knowing that it wasn't an actual option or possibility. My mother, perhaps, had the best suggestion; "Talk to your union and tell them the assignments you're taking. Also document that you don't feel safe or comfortable taking these assignments." Out of all the suggestions I took my older sister's advice— *Work Harder.* I was hoping they would give me some nugget of wisdom or the concrete solution, but just like anything else in life, it was never that simple. I kept plugging away, hoping I could please God. I decided more prayer would help.

I had fallen off with my Alcohol Support Group meetings significantly—I was only making one a week online at best. I had made one single in-person meeting over the winter in the back yard of a group member I'd never met, around a fire, and it was delightful. I wished they could have it every night because the Zoom Alcohol Support Group could not compare to the in-person spiritual recharge and fellowship we got from attending. Regardless of meetings or phone calls made, God was always there for me and I had a direct line to Him whenever I needed. This was the power of prayer for me. He was my first and last line of defense against bad decisions and thinking like a 'NUT' —Negative Unproductive Thinking.

March 2021

Curveball!

The first two weeks of March were the same rate of short staffing. Every other day I had the extra twelve to fifteen residents. I was completely used to it by now. I worked with no break—just five minutes to shovel food down my throat and move on. I eventually decided that I would take my hour break at 11:30 and watch Netflix or soccer on the computer at my desk. They were deducting that break from my pay either way, so I had to make up for it.

They had just installed computers at all the nursing stations, as well as printers. They replaced the existing fax machines as well. They were making an effort to modernize the facility, but after two or three weeks, *all* the printers broke. They bought printers made for people's homes, for printing things once in a while. The IT person confirmed that the printers' memories were fried from all the data they were attempting to process. They still lay in the same spot where they broke. The computers worked well enough.

Shawna's vaccine tour in California was still going well and coming to an end. She enjoyed the observation nursing because it was less work than actually drawing up syringes full of the solution and shooting it into the arm of the victim. She also enjoyed talking to all the people who came through. In those fifteen minutes, she got to know people and their walk of life. Nearly everyone outside of Texas always got a kick out of where she was from, and her fun accent. It was like she was an unknown celebrity wherever she went. She'd always get the typical questions: "Do you shoot guns?" Yes. "Do you ride horses?" Of course. "Do you eat a lot of steak?" Sure do!

Eventually, Shawna had to go to Louisiana to look after her mom, who was going through some mental changes. She had to end her contract early to take care of her mother. Shawna's step-father wasn't taking care of her and her cognitive abilities were declining.

I was waiting for an update regarding the whole situation, and she called as I was getting ready for bed; "What do you think about my mom coming to live with us for a little bit?"

"Of course. That's fine." I sort of saw this coming and didn't care. We had the space in our one-bedroom loft and family was family. I didn't ask any questions about the length of stay or anything like that.

"I'm going to have to get my cousins to help move all her stuff to storage. She's not staying with that asshole anymore." Her sweet tone left and it turned to anger and frustration.

I didn't want her to elaborate and she didn't. We hung up moments later and I started to wonder what life would be like with her mom and her dog. The apartment was plenty spacious for two humans and two cats, but throw another human and another pet into the mix and it would get very small very quickly. I decided not to worry or wonder, but to trust in God that it would play out the way it was meant to.

It had been one year since COVID. I was a full nurse and pandemic nursing was my only experience. I figured I could get a job anywhere with what I had been through. I was proud to have heeded the call of duty. I still hadn't seen my friends in over a year now. I saw my family here and there around the pool, or outside for ten minutes, fifteen feet from each other in a parking lot or driveway. I saw my niece once at a summer swim at my sister and brother-in-law's new house and pool. My extended family—forget it. I still hadn't seen my brother, his wife, and their three kids during the year of COVID. I had to have faith in this vaccine and its ability to get us all back to normal.

Lucie Greer, Jeoffrey Pratt, Luna, and I continued to try and run the unit and look out for all the other two dozen residents. Everyone knew their roles, who to look out for, and when to look. Lucie always called me kid, and it always made me think of being young again and doing it all over. She told new residents and neighbors how I was always making people laugh, but when it came down to actual nursing, I was the best in the facility, and I would always get done what needed to be done and would always look out for my residents. She also told me how I should be on stage. This was something my beloved grandmother would always tell me. When she first said that, I immediately thought about my grandmother Bridget and wondered if she'd be pleased with me and my recent transformation, and the work I was doing with the elderly.

Luna bought me a Stephen King book, called "The Stand." It was a brand new, big, beautiful, hardcover book. I knew I probably shouldn't have accepted the gift but decided to "borrow" it and told her I would give it back at some point. Maybe I'd forget to give it back but I didn't worry that far in advance. I started reading it the night she gave it to me. In the foreword, it mentioned how this was one of the most popular books he had written and most loved by all his fans. The version I received had extra parts written in it because apparently, the first copy didn't have everything Mr. King wanted to include. I was touched that Luna thought of me and was excited to start a new novel. Watching sports and TV by myself was getting old.

Shawna brought her mom back to New Jersey in late March and our world was turned upside-down. She had severe dementia and it was very sad. As soon as I began to think of the future and what would happen and how we would live, my Alcohol Support Group's famous mantra rang loud in my head, *One Day At A Time*.

Once Rhianna moved in, I was exposed to dementia and caring for the elderly 24/7. I laughed about it and decided to not overthink it or stress this thing I couldn't control. Dementia was more of a monster than a thing. I had to keep the selfish thinking at bay and think about what Shawna needed from me. I needed to support her and tell her she was doing a great job and let her know that I was there for her. We decided the best place for Rhianna would be in the master bedroom with the walk-in closet that connected to the master bathroom. We would move our whole bedroom up to the loft. All our furniture and all the walk-in closet items had to go upstairs to the loft, but only about half of it actually fit.

Shawna contacted a mattress guy we'd discovered on Craigslist and she and her mom traveled fifty miles south in a rented Home Depot truck to pick up a brand new queen mattress from his storage unit. They brought the mattress back and bought a cheap bed frame from Walmart. I got back from work and Rhianna's bedroom was all but set up. Shawna couldn't return to work any time soon. She had to get all of Rhianna's Medicare and benefits transferred to Rhianna's new address. She had to find a primary doctor, get a full workup done, see what medications needed adjusting as well as new medications she would need, and get a dentist to pull some teeth. Rhianna also needed a knee replacement... and a divorce. Shawna was now a full-time personal assistant and babysitter.

My father came by to drop some things off and asked me how it was going. I told him about Rhianna's dementia and how it manifested each day. He had been going through the same things as a live-in caretaker for my grandfather for the last ten years. Suddenly my father and I could relate in a deep way.

Although COVID was practically gone, we still had to wear surgical face masks and all the residents went back to a semi-normal life inside the nursing home. There were still the staffing shortages, which meant sitting in their own waste or not getting food or water on time. The facility was still infested with mice and cockroaches. Staff members and other residents would still steal personal items, cash, and other valuables. The weekends off that the staff looked forward to, were still dreaded by the residents. They would have only their roommate and the rare visit from a CNA or Nurse. Many residents went hours without being changed or cared for. Once Monday came, the building was full of employees ready to help. Since the State only visited on weekdays they were never able to witness the war crimes that took place over the weekends.

By this point, Luna's individual weight loss had achieved new heights—or lows—on the scale. She had lost eighty-five pounds in the last five months. Not only was she doing the exercise group four or five days a week, but she was also doing weight training and cardiovascular exercise. She would do bicep curls with eight to fifteen-pound weights daily. She would also do laps in her wheelchair daily. On occasion, she would hit a hundred laps in a full day. Each lap was eight-hundredths of a mile, bringing her total to eight miles! Her transformation and transition into fitness were remarkable. She eventually started to walk again. She would walk much smaller laps with her buddy Henry Potter following behind her with her wheelchair in case she had to sit down quickly. Seeing them work together would get even the coldest of hearts all warm and fuzzy. Luna lost these eighty-five pounds in spite of her daunting primary diagnoses of Chronic

Kidney Disease, Diabetes, Hypertension, *and* Multiple Sclerosis! I shared the news, just like I did the 90-year-old COVID survivors, to anyone with two ears. I then liked to ask my audience, "What's *your* excuse?" Due to her weight loss, she stopped needing insulin altogether! She also became continent of bladder, waking up to a dry bed most mornings. Anything really is possible!

I worked on a new bit which I was particularly proud of, even though it was not impressive or skillful at all: While the exercise group was on break outside of Leslie Dawson's, I would start the magic show. "Good evening, Ladies and Gentlemen! My name is the great Davini! I will show you how I can disappear before your very eyes!" I put my best showman hat on, puffing out my chest and doing my best to imitate a circus frontman. Many of the residents rolled their eyes and I heard Tabatha say, *Oh, God*—but I ignored her like I always did when she would try to rain on my parade—or circus, in this case.

"Here we have a very ordinary door!" I started knocking on Leslie's large door, testing the handle, "May I have a volunteer from the crowd, please!? Ah yes. You'll do, Sir!" I took Henry Potter by the hand (because he was the only one in the bunch who could walk) and led him a couple of paces to the door. "Please inspect the door and make sure there are no holes, or smoke or mirrors." Henry was extremely confused but did his best. "I'm going to disappear from behind that door in five seconds!" I tried to make eye contact with everyone, knowing that I was losing their attention quickly. "Okay, I will disappear into the thin air before your eyes! Henry! Open this door in five seconds!"

He nodded but I wasn't sure he'd be able to follow through... I went in and closed the door. I opened the bathroom door and went through to Tabatha's connecting room, and waited... I heard that Luna was the only one counting... I slowly cracked Tabatha's door and looked and could see that Henry had opened the door. I pulled the door open and jumped out with both hands in the air. "Aha! The great Davini has done it again! Magic before your very eyes! But don't ask me how, for I shall *never* reveal my powers!"

As with any bit I did, some would laugh, some would wonder what happened and Tabatha would surely try to ruin all the fun.

"You... went... through... the... bathroo-" she stated slowly and agitated.

"I. Shall. Never! Reveal my powers!" Laughing out loud I got back to my med-cart. At least I enjoyed the bit and patted myself on the back for my elementary wit. I looked to my left and Henry was still in Leslie's room looking through the bathroom, maybe he was looking for snacks. This made it all worth it.

"All right, all right, back to exercising. We gotta work for that dinner tonight! Let's get it going!" I started clapping as even Luna was rolling her eyes, but taking her position to get everyone pumping again. It was the little moments like this that made me happy. I wasn't a real entertainer but I'm sure I brought some amount of joy and entertainment to them, even if they just thought I was silly or crazy. None of the other nurses were doing magic tricks, I could guarantee that.

Another favorite bit was taking a picture of a baby from a magazine and gluing it onto a popsicle stick. I would then walk into everyone's rooms and hold it in front of my face and start crying like a baby. No matter the cognitive level, *every* resident couldn't help but to laugh hysterically. This bit had the highest batting average and I loved to hear everyone laugh.

Gratuity List

I still think to this day how COVID was a blessing to me and how fortunate I was to have all the events of my life play out the way I did. COVID provided a stressful, scary, high-stakes setting for the beginning of my career. Nothing in the rest of my nursing career would ever compare to it—it was my measuring stick and surely it could only get better from there on out. If another pandemic did come, I would be prepared, having already lived and worked through one. Even in the crazy and hectic environment COVID provided, there was still a sense of no pressure since everyone was expected to die at the beginning and we could only do our best. It was like when a team was getting blown out and the less experienced players came in because at that point it didn't matter.

I was compensated well financially for my duties. I always thought I could have gotten more compared to what others were receiving, but at the end of the day I was extremely happy with what I *did* get.

I got to meet dozens of new people from all over the country. I still keep in touch with a handful of them through social media. Thanks to the traveling nurses and CNAs, I learned much more about healthcare and nursing than I ever would have from my set regulars at my facility.

I got to meet Shawna, the love of my life. Many people never even hit the lottery once. I hit the lottery once when I got sober, and then again when I met Shawna. We were pretty much the same person. We had huge hearts but were fierce when we needed to be. We were physically and mentally tough. We loved having fun and living outside the rules. We never stressed the small stuff and were always grateful. We also loved the gym. I'll say it again: *excercise*. It keeps us healthy, but more importantly for me it keeps me happy and keeps my head in the right space. I   am grateful for Alcohol Support Groups and the relationship with my Higher

Power it is responsible for. I am also grateful Shawna also loves to come to my Alcohol Support Groups and meeting my glum group's members.

I am grateful that none of my family member's or friend's health were directly affected by COVID.

I am grateful I am healthy to continue to try and make a difference in the world at every level.

Conclusion

The COVID did at least give all the residents a talking point for most likely the rest of their lives in there. I tried my best to bring joy and happiness every day I came. I thought that, because I'd gotten sober, my residents pretty much got the best version of me each day I showed up for work. If I had been drinking I would have been hung over. If I'd been hung over I would have automatically been in a foul mood. If I'd been in a foul mood these residents wouldn't get any joy, or receive any love—only medications. I would be the staff member who would finish their half-assed work early and sit down and couldn't be bothered.

Without Alcohol Support Groups and the faith in God I rediscovered from them, there would be no rebirth for me. There would be no COVID nurse in me. I could barely take care of myself, let alone twenty-seven elderly residents battling every disease we ever learned about in nursing school. I thought about how brilliant God was and how long He might have been planning my transcendence and development into a functioning, hardworking, and reliable member of society. I thanked Him for all the adversity I encountered each day. I thanked Him for the opportunity for growth. I thanked Him for all my blessings. Turning your life around is possible. God and faith played and continue to play a big part in my 180. Anything is possible one day at a time.

I finally realized the foremost important trait that the nurse must possess in order to succeed in the grueling healthcare industry—a big heart. As long as the nurse has a big heart full of compassion the rest will surely follow.

Wash your hands and check your blood pressure, and Always be of service to others.

Thank you for letting me share!

Printed in the United States
by Baker & Taylor Publisher Services